MW01169746

Your Child Doesn't Have To Die!

How you can help your child overcome
cancer with nutritional therapy

Leanne Sorteberg
with Lisa C. Ragsdale

Published by
Abundant Living
P.O. Box 1092, Burnsville, MN   55337
E-mail   abundliv@aol.com

ISBN 0-9654714-0-3

Printed by Ideal Printers, Inc., St. Paul, MN

The information in this book is not a substitute for medical advice.
There is no guarantee that following the protocol outlined in this book
will have the same results with everyone. The publisher and authors are
not responsible for any effects or consequences resulting from the use of
nutritional therapy as outlined in this book. Our purpose is to make
nutritional therapy as an option known to the public.   Anyone
considering a protocol of nutritional therapy as an option in treating
cancer should do so under the supervision of a network of health
professionals.

"As the heavens are higher than the earth, so are my ways higher than your ways and my thoughts than your thoughts. As the rain and the snow come down from heaven, and do not return to it without watering the earth and making it bud and flourish, so that it yields seed for the sower and bread for the eater, so is my word that goes out from my mouth: It will not return to me empty, but will accomplish what I desire and achieve the purpose for which I sent it."

Isaiah 55:9-11 (NIV)

Contents

Book II: Key Points of Nutritional Therapy For Cancer

Dedication

*This book is dedicated to my Lord Jesus
Christ, and to my six children, all of whom
continued to love me when I was unlovable.*

*Jeff
Jake
Aubree
Andrew
Luke
&
Lauren*

Acknowledgements

How much to be prized and esteemed is a friend,
On whom we may always with safety depend;
Our joys when extended will always increase,
And griefs when divided are hushed into peace.

Needles and Friends, from Friendship's Offering by Susan McKelvey

This book would still be swimming around in my head if it weren't for the writing ability of my sister, Lisa Ragsdale. Lisa, thanks for your time, effort, and energy. I know producing this book took all three from you. Thank God for B-complex! You've continued to inspire me in my life. Sacrifices were made by your family as well. Thanks for your patience Tim, Jenna, Leslye, Jonathan and Keith. I am indebted to you and I love you all.

Humbly and happily I express my gratitude to the authors, doctors and nutritionists I've learned from. The Frahms, the Balches, Danny Vierra, Paul Barry, Dr. Wurdemann and his wife, Lisa. Thank you for paving the way so that simple people like me can "dig in" to the truths that you so eloquently share.

Thank you to the supporters and encouragers at Valley Natural Foods, always willing to answer one last question.

Thank you to my family and friends who stood by us during those dark days and allow us today to filter out the pain of our experiences by talking and sometimes crying it out.

Thank you to our "angel" Debbie Murphy, because Andrew "sees the sun when it rains." He feels "like an ice cube when it's ninety-five and humid." He colors rainbows and flowers in the wintertime. You've influenced our young son by your positive attitude. I see your spirit daily in his life.

Thank You to all the friends that did extradordinary things for me, who were there for me during this trial, and who continued to accept me when my behavior was unacceptable.

Kelly Abrahamian
Sue Bird
Joy Havlik
Jeanne Inkala
Margaret Johnson
Michelle Minea
Marcy Munson
Debbie Murphy
Gail Schultz
Elizabeth Shults
Theresa Tykeson
Lisa Wurdemann

And to my wonderful husband, David, your willingness to allow me to be myself is a gift more precious than jewels. Thank you for all you have sacrificed to make this book a reality.

*Finally, I'm grateful to you, the reader. As you hold this book and read its contents, may your heart and mind be opened to God's truths concerning healing our bodies **and** our souls. I pray that these simple words will make a difference in yet another life.*

Preface

The Sortebergs live in Burnsville, MN with their six children. Four of the six children, including Andrew have birth defects that doctors believe to be associated with Leanne's use of the drug Accutane under the advice of a dermatologist shortly after her first child was born.

Leanne's first child Jeff, was born a normal, healthy baby in July of 1985. In 1987 Leanne married David Sorteberg and their first child Jake was born the next year. Jake had serious birth defects. He was diagnosed with Total Anomalous Pulmonary Venus return to the Coronary Sinus and also a "micro-stomach". His stomach was too small to hold the nourishment that he needed in order to grow. He required three open heart surgeries, a total of nine surgeries on his chest and abdomen which left his body extremely vulnerable to disease. A gastrostomy was done so that he could be fed continuously through a tube going directing into his small stomach. The tube, called a G-tube, is referred to in this story. Jake endured numerous bouts of pneumonia. He needed essential supplemental oxygen until he was four and a half, and he was attached to a feed pump for the first five years of his life.

The Sorteberg's second child is a girl, Aubree, who was diagnosed at the age of 15 months with mitral valve stenosis which can be corrected by a fairly common procedure called angioplasty.

Andrew is their third child together. He was born in June of 1991. He had health problems relating to his diet almost immediately and finally at the age of 18 months he was diagnosed with a Stage IV neuroblastoma. This is a very deadly form of childhood cancer. There was little hope for his recovery, nor for restoration of the quality of life that every child should enjoy. Through months of grueling treatments, tests and hospital stays, this family endured much physical and emotional pain and exhaustion.

Left nearly hopeless after eleven months of rigid chemotherapy and radiation treatments, the Sortebergs believe that God led them to wholly pursue nutritional therapy for treatment of Andrew's grave illness. In this endeavor, they were advised and supported by a network of doctors and specialists while spending many hours personally researching the benefits and methods of nutritional healing.

Their story here is written for two reasons: To proclaim the good works of God in their lives and to illustrate how His presence was displayed throughout their trial. And to educate others that nutritional therapy is a viable alternative even for such devastating diseases as childhood cancers.

There is a purpose for the pain Andrew and his family endured. People always wonder how a loving God can allow children to suffer. Leanne always asked the Lord "Why did my sons, Jake and Andrew have to suffer so much?" She would not accept that it was simply to refine her character and make her a better person. That concept offended her and just made her feel worse, because she thought, "I must be an awful person because my children have to suffer terribly so I will change." But that's not it. There is a higher purpose for their pain than just making better human beings out of them. Now, when Leanne is out there speaking in front of people about the experiences and the suffering of her children, hearts begin to open and tears start to fall. That's what the suffering of innocent children does. It opens hearts to consider a better way. Not only a better way to approach cancer, but a better way to approach life, in humble dependence upon the Creator who made us. He is the one who made our bodies and the resources in this earth to heal them. Ultimately, He deserves all the glory for Andrew's victory.

Leanne knows now why God allowed her children to suffer. Hearts need to be broken open and it's painful. As people hear of Andrew's suffering through chemo and radiation treatments, they become open and anxious to hear how this little boy's life was saved. They become willing to consider nutritional therapy as a serious option for life after disease, and to consider God's option for eternal life that is open to all of us who believe in him. When she sees tears in the eyes of a crowd she tells them, "I see now why the Lord allowed my children to suffer, it's there in your eyes."

Throughout Andrew's recovery, Leanne has felt called to be an advocate for nutritional therapy and to share with people the lessons that her family has learned in fighting his cancer. She shares key points on diet, how to try to maintain a healthy emotional life, and positive attitude through an intimate relationship with the Lord. Her hope for the reader, is that these pages will be enlightening and encourage a further investigation of nutritional therapy for the health of your body, and about seeking God's guidance for the well-being of your soul. Her prayer for you is that you would allow God to lead you as he has led her and her husband in Andrew's struggle with cancer. Whatever physical or spiritual problem you have, the Sortebergs hope that God would give you an unquenchable thirst for health and spiritual wellness after reading their story.

1

Andrew's First Year:Foreboding symptoms

I didn't notice any particular problems during my pregnancy with Andrew other than a fall that occurred when I was seven months along. I was leaving the house to take a babysitter home one winter night. It was dark and the back steps were covered with ice. I slipped and fell down four concrete steps onto the icy walkway. I landed right on my tailbone. I stayed there for about 15-20 minutes on the ice because I was afraid to move and it hurt. My kids were screaming. My husband, David stayed there and talked to me until I felt like I could get up and move. Eventually, I was able to get up and start moving around.

The fall that I had when I was seven months pregnant, just didn't seem that significant to me and Andrew was born in June of 1991 without any problems. However, seven days after he was born, I had what I thought were labor pains all over again. We had been sitting on the couch watching a movie and they came on very fast. I began screaming in pain. I was trying the breathing techniques for labor and David was there holding my hand. I was in intense pain and it lasted for three or four hours. Just as we were getting ready to go to the emergency room it stopped. My bleeding stopped then too. I thought maybe I had a bloodclot and I called the doctor. She assured me that I would be fine, and I shouldn't worry, so I didn't think much more of it.

I nursed Andrew for about four months, nevertheless, he had problems with reflux very early on. His food would come back up after every feeding. We switched his formulas a half-dozen times either to soy or other brand names, but he continued to spit up and we thought some medication might help. Our doctor put him on Reglan, which is a drug for gastro-esophageal reflux. Our second eldest son, Jake had been on that, so we requested that it be prescribed for Andrew, thinking it was just a problem with our boys. They did a couple of tests to see if there was any obstruction and didn't find anything. At the age of six months, he was on medication to control his excessive spitting up.

In April of 1992 the house we were renting was sold. Fortunately, we were able to move in with our friends, Mark and Michelle Minea. Andrew got a cold then, and I remember thinking, "You know, he's under stress. We are moving into this strange house and David has started school full-time and is working full-time." It was early in my pregnancy with my fifth child, and I was sick all the time, not able to do much. Here was this poor little eleven month old, being tossed about and wondering what's going on. I reasoned the stress of that made him sick. Now I know that a cold is the first sign that your immune system is supressed. He had what I thought was a simple virus, but he never got over it. Also, from that point on his disposition began to change.

Andrew was always pretty happy and loving, but he became fussy and irritable most of the time. He was also a very poor eater, so if I could get anything into him I would. Unfortunately, it was typically a dairy product. (If I had known what I know now about dairy products, I never would have done it.) I would give him yogurt, or anything smooth and creamy that he liked. We were having hard times financially then, so instead of buying him formula, I gave him whole milk in his bottle. It was the worst thing I could possibly do for him but, that's a whole other chapter...

Despite our efforts to medicate him and feed him soothing foods, he continued to spit up. When he would eat a meal, we were so glad and felt we could relax some. Then all of a sudden it would come oozing back out all over his highchair tray. It was so frustrating. We had no idea what was going on. I took him to the doctor in June when he was a year old. I told my pediatrician I was really concerned about him. I talked about Andrew with her during that appointment, but I'd taken Aubree in also. Aubree had pulmonary valve stenosis and that was the year they were going to do the angioplasty on her heart. So my pediatrician was preoccupied with listening to Aubree's heart while I was throwing all these different symptoms at her about Andrew. She and I look back now, and we see what a mistake that was, because if she hadn't been so focused on Aubree, maybe she would have heard more specifically what I was telling her about Andrew. I don't blame her for being in tune to Aubree, and I'm glad that she was, because her condition is serious too. It's something that I trust the Lord about because it's useless to look back and wonder "what if". I believe that for some divine reason, it was God's ultimate plan for that day. We went home from that appointment and Andrew continued to struggle all through the summer. He threw up his food all the time. He was irritable, fussy, and whiney, and very difficult for us to cope with.

That summer, we lived with our friends, the Minea's, and the Havlich's, and David's parents. The house we had been renting was being sold and we weren't able to find another place we could afford for some time. We even lived at my parent's primitive cabin for a little while. Finally, in August of 1992 we moved into a two-bedroom apartment with our four children, Jeff, Jake, Aubree and Andrew. I was in the middle of my fifth pregnancy. Although we were thrilled about having our own place, we were still bothered with Andrew's relentless spitting up.

In October I took Andrew to the doctor again and recited all the same frustrating symptoms to her. I said, "Something is wrong, something is going on." Once again, she didn't see anything and she didn't feel the need to investigate his symptoms at that time. I couldn't help feeling like she wasn't listening to me. Unfortunately, she was going through breast cancer at the time, and this kept her from fully concentrating on Andrew's symptoms.

During the next couple of months things got worse. Dealing with Andrew got more aggravating, and more frustrating. Finally, I was talking to a friend about his symptoms and I realized that it was a serious problem. I laid it all out on the table with someone who could look at it objectively and she said, "You've got to do something."

I scheduled an appointment for Andrew again. This time I had an actual list of his symptoms on paper, because I wanted the doctor to go through that list, look at everything I'd written down and find an explanation for it. The appointment was scheduled for a Monday and they called and cancelled because our doctor had something going on. I was disappointed, because I wanted her to be there. She had been seeing Andrew for that whole year.

On Wednesday that week as I was changing Andrew's diaper, I noticed what I thought was a hiatal hernia. There was a large lump protruding from his groin area. I thought, "There! That's it! That's the problem." I was so relieved, because I thought it was something that could be easily corrected. When I called the doctor's office, they said he wasn't in any danger but to bring him in that day. I was informed that our doctor wasn't in then and would be back on Monday. I told them, "She's been dealing with us all along and if there is really no concern then I want to wait until she's going to be there." So we waited through the weekend.

That Saturday I was driving to a women's retreat with a friend, and I told her, "I don't know, tell me if I'm paranoid, but I think something awful is going to happen. I've got my guard up and I'm expecting the worst. I'm expecting them to tell us that it is a hiatal hernia and they'll have to do surgery, and Andrew's going to be in the hospital right when I'm due with Luke, and when we're due to move. I just know it's going to happen all at once. Do you think I'm paranoid?" My friend answered, "No, I think you're just being a realist." Little did I know what awful news was to come.

2

"We've found a large mass..."

The following Monday was our appointment, but our pediatrician had been called out for an emergency. Dr. Ross Olson, who is a wonderful Christian doctor examined Andrew. He asked David and I a lot of questions. I showed him my list and he looked at it. I kept that list in my purse for a long time after Andrew was diagnosed. Now we keep it in Andrew's "special box" of momentos. Dr. Olson examined Andrew very thoroughly. He's not a man of many words, and he didn't say very much during the examination. Then he walked abruptly out of the room.

David and I sat there looking at each other feeling like we had not even been noticed. It must have taken him about 15 minutes to come back in, but he came back in with our pediatrician who we'd been told was across town. She walked right over to Andrew and examined him. As they turned around and looked at us, I knew they were scared to death to say something. There was a stern hardness about them, a facade of forced strength, but I could see past it to the fear. I had seen the same look in the doctor's eyes who told us about Jake's condition at birth. They said, "We have found a large mass in his abdomen. It appears to be grapefruit-sized or larger, and we would like to schedule an ultrasound. It could be one of three things: It could be a cancerous tumor, a benign tumor, or a very rare disorder which is highly unlikely." I cannot describe how we felt at that moment. Certainly, panic began to well up inside of me, yet my mind was instantly shifting into a survival mode. I wanted to know what we could do next, where we were supposed to go from there. David and I managed to quietly agree that an ultrasound made sense. We didn't panic outwardly, but were anxious to find out what this was as soon as possible.

They wanted us to have some x-rays taken right then and some more bloodwork. I knew then, that it was going to be longer than we expected, so I went out to make a phone call to my friend Elizabeth who was watching our other children. I said, "Elizabeth, they found a large mass in Andrew's abdomen." And then for the first time, I *lost it*. I was crying and screaming at the same time. I sobbed, "Will you watch the kids? Will you call the pastors? Will you get people praying for us?" In that first moment alone with this information it had settled in and I panicked.

After I had regained my composure I went back into the exam room. Shakily, we went about our business getting his tests and bloodwork done. The doctors couldn't schedule an ultrasound for that afternoon, because it was already after 5 p.m., so they scheduled the next available time which was Wednesday, two days away. We agreed on that and were allowed to go home.

When we were leaving the doctors office, all the nurses were still there and they all tried to say something supportive. I could sense that they were crushed by the doctors' discovery too. These nurses had been through everything with Jake from the time we moved back to Minnesota from Colorado where he was born. They were in awe over this devastating news about yet another of our children.

David and I were in some kind of shock. I don't remember he and I talking to one another. I just remember that we would look at each other and we would look at Andrew. It seemed like everything he did was so precious and so much more adorable than before this frightening news. On the way home in our van, an exhausted Andrew had fallen asleep right away. We were driving down the freeway and simultaneously David and I started to sing one of our favorite songs: "God will make a way, when there seems to be no way. He works in ways we cannot see. He will make a way for me." It was so strange for us to start singing at the same time because we weren't even looking at each other. We were both looking straight ahead. Then we both started crying and then smiled to tell each other, "Yeah, God's going to make a way."

As we exited the interstate Andrew woke up and said, "French fries", which was his favorite food. We said, "You betcha buddy!" and we stopped and bought Andrew some supper at a fast-food place. We sat there in the restaraunt not saying much to each other but adoring what he did, even if he fussed, we adored it. We silently appreciated his priceless, now so vulnerable, little life. Anyone watching us that evening, playing and talking with Andrew, would never have known that anything was wrong. Yet inside Andrew, there was a deadly cancer, determined to consume him, and inside of me, a fear that grew like cancer threatening to explode.

Jake was still being fed with his G-tube and sometime between Monday and Wednesday it fell out. What a nuisance that was. We decided to save a trip and schedule putting his G-tube back in on Wednesday at the same time Andrew's ultrasound was going on. We went in for the ultrasound, which was quite an extensive one. When it was finished, the doctors and the radiologist told us, "Yes, this is in fact a very large mass, it appears to be cancerous, but we can't say for sure. We will have to do a biopsy. We are talking to the surgeons right now to see when they can schedule the surgery. It should be done soon as possible."

We barely had time to react when they announced they were ready for Jake in the ER to have his tube placed. David took Andrew to the playroom and my Mom came with me and Jake to the ER. Jake was lying on the table, and we were talking to the doctors about what type of tube we wanted. As the doctors began inserting the tube, blood suddenly began squirting out of Jake's abdomen. He started screaming and nurses had to come to hold him down. He yelled at me to make them stop, and I tried to tell him that it was a good thing, that we needed to feed him and this was the best way. I told him we loved him, and did my best to calm him down.

Our gastrologist walked in and tried to manipulate Jake's abdomen to take the tube. It was difficult because it had been out for a day and a half. He looked at me and realized I was extremely pregnant. I could tell he was wondering if I would be alright. Just as he looked at me, another doctor walked in and said, "Hi Mrs. Sorteberg, I'm Glen Anderson, I'm the surgeon for your son Andrew and I would like to schedule surgery with you at eight in the morning on Friday. Could you be admitted Thursday night or afternoon for pre-op? We can do a biopsy Friday morning."   I said, "That's fine."   And he said, "OK, great, see you then."   He walked out of the room and Dr. Stafford, the gastrologist struggling to put the tube in Jake, looked at my mom and said, "Oh, my God."   Then he looked at me and then back at my mom again.   He said, "Is she going to be OK?"   My mom answered, "Oh yeah, she'll be OK."   And you know, I was OK--on the outside. I had to be OK. I had to be strong. Jake needed me then, and I couldn't respond or react to anything else. On the inside though, I really wasn't OK, and months later all that stored up emotion exploded on me.

Jake's tube eventually got placed and we headed home.   It was late on Wednesday night and we were going admit Andrew to the hospital Thursday evening. We called friends and family, to announce what was going on and asked them for prayer. I told David that I wanted to go to the mall and get some decent clothes, because I would be at the hospital and around people. I was in the last month of my pregnancy and had just one pair of pants to wear and two shirts.

We had been together that whole chaotic week at appointments. When I got up on Thursday morning and went to the mall, I was suddenly alone. I drove no more than a half-mile away from our home before I lost it again. A song by Leslie Phillips was playing in the car stereo, "The Strength of My Life."   When I heard it I totally fell apart.   I was bawling, and sobbing uncontrollably to the point where I had to pull over and I couldn't drive. I didn't know what to do and I was crying so hard that I was screaming. I couldn't make myself stop. I felt paralyzed, and I didn't think I could possibly regain composure enough to drive. I was afraid that I would be stuck there, parked by the side of the road crying. The song ended and I shut the stereo off. I continued to drive wiping my tears and taking deep breaths. I told myself, " I have to get these clothes and get back home and get ready to go to the hospital." But when I got to the parking lot, I did it again.   I started screaming and crying again. I cried out, "God help us!" and "I'm scared!" Physically, my body was letting all its stress out and it seemed like I wasn't emotionally there. I know now, that I was grieving the loss of my life as I had known it. I had done the same thing with Jake. I had been suddenly thrust into a nightmare the night he was born and I didn't have a healthy little baby boy to take home. I had the constant anxiety of surgeries, medicines, and life and death decisions. Just as I was beginning to awaken and live a somewhat stable life with Jake, I was plunged again into the nightmarish world of cancer with Andrew. I was not only very scared for my son and what he was about to go through, but I was also mourning the loss of what was supposed to be. Jake had survived and we all expected that everyone would be healthy and happy and we could move on to better days.

Finally, I was able to walk into the mall and I remember a lady looking at me as if she thought, "Oh my gosh, she looks like she's been through hell and back." I quickly picked out some things, paid for them and left. I drove across the street to a department store because we needed diapers and some other things for Andrew's hospital stay. The next thing I knew, a lady grabbed me by the arm and led me to another lady who was an employee of the store. One of them said, "Ma'am you are standing in the hallway turning circles. Can we help you?" I said, "I came here..." and then I stopped and they asked, "Are you lost? Are you looking for something?" I said, "I came here to get something." They helped me try to remember what I came for. Then I realized it was diapers. I went to get them and I was on my way.

Before I left the store, I called my friend, Jeanne. I said, "I'm in trouble. I've got to get in the car again and I can't drive and I'm scared." She said, "Just stay right there and I'll come to get you." I told her, "No, I've got to make it. I have to get through this. I have a couple days that I need to be ready for and I've just got to get through this." She was in tears on the other end of the phone because she wanted to be there with me so badly. I said, "I don't want to be alone, and I'm going to go back to the apartment. Everyone's gone and I can't be alone and I'm scared, because I'm falling apart when I'm alone. Will you be there when I get there?" She promised me that and I started to leave, but I couldn't leave the parking lot because I started crying again. I knew that I could not continue to be alone. I cried all the way back home. Sure enough, Jeanne met me there and I calmed down. It was good to have someone to talk to, to distract me and to keep me busy. Being close to the family, Jeanne was upset about Andrew's illness too, and it helped me to be able to comfort her. The conversation kept my mind occupied while we did laundry and prepared for the hospital stay.

3

Diagnosis:Stage IV Neuroblastoma

When David came home we went to the hospital, leaving our other children with friends. That night family and some friends came to Andrew's room to visit. He was so adorable. We took some pictures of him and then everybody had to leave. David and I were alone again, just looking at each other not knowing what to say. We met new nurses and hospital staff and looked at each other shaking our heads and questioning, "Can you believe this? Can you believe we are here all over again, yet it's another child. What if this is cancerous?" And we comforted each other with the knowledge that this time, we knew the Lord.

As we were getting ready to go to bed that night, something really stupid happened. David went into the bathroom to wash his hands. He had just taken his glasses off, because we were getting into bed. As he pushed down on the chemical soap dispenser, it squirted in his eye. Here it was eleven o'clock at night and they ended up having to write up a big report because the soap can cause blindness if it gets in your eyes. David had to go over to Abbott-Northwestern Hospital which adjoins Minneapolis Children's and be examined in the ER. We thought, "Boy, this is ridiculous. Just one more thing on top of all this. Jake's G-tube was enough, but this was getting ridiculous." He came back and we tried to get some sleep that night.

Everyone was there that Friday morning for the surgery. My brother, Mike and his wife, Jeri were there. My sister, Lynn and my mom and dad were there. Our pastors

Mark and Doug were there. We were such a large group that we were told to wait in an outer lobby.

It was so hard to let Andrew go into surgery. All I could think was, "Here I go again, he's absolutely adorable, cute and smiling, and soon he will be screaming in pain. And I'm letting it happen. I'm signing the papers to give them permission to do it to him." Putting a child into surgery is the greatest fear that I have ever known. It is heartbreaking to know that this little boy who can be cuddled and warm in your arms will soon be cut open with cold steel. He will be in so much pain, having tubes coming out of his body every which way. And we knew that once we surrendered him, we might not get him back. It is the ugliest feeling I have ever experienced.

Andrew was taken into surgery Friday morning, December 10, 1992. We waited for what seemed like a long time. It actually took about three or four hours. It was an intense wait, because we would learn if the tumor was cancerous or not. Of course, we were all silently praying that it wouldn't be. It was exciting to have our pastors there around our family members that were unbelievers. My dad took a liking to Mark, so that was neat. We sat and we talked, but pretty much everyone paced around and glanced at each other now and then like people do when they wait for bad news.

Finally the doctor came and he sat down with David and I. Everyone was tense. He started telling us that they had biopsied the tumor five times and found it to be malignant and that Andrew's condition was serious. It was very large and they were unable to remove it because it had finger-like tentacles attached to Andrew's kidneys and liver. They had found cancer in his bone marrow, too. All of us were stunned and did not even try to hold back our emotions. My mom was sobbing. My brother and his wife were crying. I sat there for the longest time crying and sobbing. David and I did not want to believe that this was happening to us. I tried to talk, asking "What are we going to do?" Again, I cried so hard, I screamed. My whole body hurt and my eyes were swollen for days. The pressure of the last few days had built up a tidal wave of fear that came crashing over me, suffocating me with pain, and paralyzing my thoughts.

While we waited for Andrew to come out of recovery, we were taken to the lab and were allowed to look at the biopsy. It looked like pink flesh. I remember feeling that this thing we were examining was evil. This small piece of flesh was eating away at my precious little blonde-haired boy.

Andrew was taken up to his room and we were able to go up to the floor with him. It was very hard to see him knowing that he had this deadly cancer raging inside of him. He was just a sweet, bubbly little boy before surgery and all of a sudden he was in incredible pain and we knew the truth, that he was gravely ill. When I was around him, I got stronger. I realized that he needed me. I had brought the tape of Leslie Phillips with me and I played it all the time. I even played it for my dad, explaining, "This is where I'm going to get my strength." He graciously listened to the whole tape and I was glad that in the midst of this terrible situation, I could share my faith in the Lord with him.

We were being told minute-by-minute what we needed to do and expect. We were being introduced to the hospital floor, the oncology floor and the nurses there. Then Andrew started having a drug-reaction to his pain meds. He actually started hallucinating. I asked the nurse, "Why is he flinging his arms like that?" And she said, "Typically, we believe that children see bugs flying before them or something flying at them." So David stretched his whole body across Andrew's, because he was thrashing so violently. He had all these tubes sticking out of him and we needed to protect him.

David wanted me to go home because I wasn't getting any sleep on the little cots we were given at the hospital. I would lay there bawling because it was so uncomfortable and I was so pregnant. I couldn't leave Andrew. It was late at night, about 11 p.m. David had left the room. He was getting frustrated because he didn't know if I was going to leave or not. I couldn't decide so he went to get a cup of coffee and sit in the parent's lounge. I was alone with Andrew who was having a hard time falling asleep. My sister, Lynn, had given me a cassette tape single with "I Will Always Love You" sung by Whitney Houston. I put it in the tape player and as I was contemplating trying to leave the hospital, I picked up Andrew and held him in my arms. As the song played I began to slow dance with him. I let my tears fall freely as we danced, in the dark room dimly lit with the lights of the monitors attached to Andrew. My whole body ached with love and pain for him. I couldn't do anything for him but love him and I couldn't let him go. I played the song three times before I set him down to sleep. I didn't leave that night. David and I both stayed.

It was an exhausting night. It was awful to watch Andrew, a sweet, smiling little boy, turned into this drugged-up little patient with this lethal mass growing inside his little body. The next few days were full of cards, phone calls, and people from church dropping in all day long. Meals were dropped off for us and people were organizing things for the other children. The wound of Andrew's diagnosis was soothed with the love and the support of people around us who pulled together in so many practical ways to help. I knew that God was going to be with us. Through His grace and mercy I was drawn to depend on him, and his peace and strength sustained me during those first emotional days. However, as time wore on, I began to rely on myself more and I began to feel that my family and I were being ripped apart at the seams.   At eighteen months of age our son Andrew was diagnosed with Stage IV neuroblastoma. Stage Four is the worst stage of cancer. Neuroblastoma is a very rare childhood cancer affecting infants and children up to ten years of age. It usually stems from the nervous system and is one of the deadliest cancers. A grapefruit-sized tumor was found in his abdomen. It was encasing his aorta, his inferior vena cava, and his mesenteric artery. It also had finger-like tentacles that were attached to his liver, kidneys and spine. It could not be removed by surgery. Cancer cells were also detected in his bone marrow. That day our oncologist assured us that Andrew's cancer was in no way a reflection of something we had done, but could give us little hope for Andrew's recovery.

4

No options: Starting conventional therapy

Our oncologist had scheduled a conference with David and I and my parents offered to come with us. We all went in and she told we had two options; traditional chemotherapy and radiation or no treatment at all. She then informed us that with treatment Andrew had less than a 25% chance of survival, and that if we chose to do nothing, he would have six months to live. If we decided to do chemo and radiation, it would be very rigorous. It would be one of the most intense programs that they offer, and it would last at least eleven months. Also, they were considering a bone marrow harvest which would have to be done in Los Angeles.

Desperate for our son's life, and believing it was our only option, we decided to go ahead with the chemotherapy and radiation. It was either that or Andrew's sure death within six months. We were given an ounce of hope, and in spite of our initial pain and confusion we clung to the hope that maybe Andrew could beat the odds.

Andrew got his first chemo at the hospital. He had been diagnosed on December 10. A week later he was started on his first dose of chemo and then we were sent home a day or two before Christmas Eve so that we could be home for the holidays. Our Christmas that year was incredible. Our church went crazy for our family. Our kids had more presents than they knew what to do with. David and I got pots and pans, sheets and blankets and towels. People had heard that David and I didn't have a watch between us, so we received five watches each! They remembered the serious health problems we had with Jake and they had been through all of that with us. They knew that we were moving into a house and that I was almost nine months pregnant. Now, Andrew was diagnosed with this terrible cancer and they wanted to show us their concern any way they could.

We came home before Christmas and Andrew actually felt better. We were told that he would feel better because typically, when cancer patients first get a dose of chemotherapy it stuns the cancer, so the patient actually feels good for the first couple of treatments. That's exactly what happened in Andrew's case. Basically, Andrew would have chemo at the hospital for one week, go home for about a week, and would have to return to be admitted for the rest of the month because of low blood cell counts. We called that "bottoming out", and sometimes, Andrew would have a blood transfusion to counteract the low counts.

We began to see typical things that happen with people on chemotherapy. Andrew's hair started coming out in clumps. It looked so awful, I couldn't wait for it all to fall out. Someone had brought him a little denim hat and he wore that the entire time that he was going through the chemo and radiation. Then he began to get really sick. He would throw up three to five times a day. One time, during this stage, Jake and Aubree both got the flu at the same time, so we literally had three ice cream buckets handy. I remember David and I running across the room trying to get there fast enough. It was gross, and very exhausting.

It was hard to focus on our other kids. I didn't have control over the choices I wanted to make as a mother. I was in the middle of homeschooling Jeff in his second grade year. It was critical time for teaching him to read. He and I had struggled with it the previous year, so I had a lot of goals and hopes for him that all fell to the wayside with Andrew's diagnosis and treatments. I was very humbled, but asked my friend, Gail to finish homeschooling him for the rest of the year. She was faithful and Jeff did learn how to read.

The disease controlled what I did. The condition and treatment of the diseased person literally affects every aspect of your life. Sometimes new parents will ask me, "You've had six children, what can we expect?" I say, "Well, you can expect that before you do, say or think anything, you have to consider that child first. You *always* have to think of them first." Inevitably, they look at me kind of dumbfounded, but it's the truth. That truth was multiplied for us with Andrew going through cancer treatment. We had to think of all of our children, but even before them, we had to put Andrew's needs first.

5

When it Rains, it Pours

The end of December was actually pretty nice, because the first round of chemo stunned the cancer enough so that we could focus on Andrew. We had a little reprieve from the intensity of the earlier days of that month, but I could hear the distant thunder of an approaching "storm." We were getting ready to move into a new home and we were hoping for everything to continue to go smoothly. We didn't know what to expect, so we took it day by day. We were packing, and there were people helping us pack. People helped us clean the apartment out, and people from our church helped us clean our new house before we moved in. Yes, the wind was definitely picking up.

Then the rain came. My doctor had a concern about my pregnancy, so she asked me to go in for an ultrasound. It happened to be scheduled the day before we were to move. Jake had double-pneumonia and we had a home health nurse taking care of him in a friend's home. I was on the phone talking with doctors trying to get Jake's medication and a nebulizer to set things up for him there. A home health nurse who is a good friend of ours said she would volunteer to give Jake's treatments and to check on him. At least there was an umbrella over Jake.

That night the storm grew worse. David and I and Andrew were alone at home. All of our kids were being taken care of by friends. Andrew's breathing started getting really labored. We called the hospital and told them about Andrew and they thought that he might have pneumonia. A friend came and picked up David and Andrew to take them to the hospital. I was ill and hadn't had much sleep, yet I had to report for my ultrasound in the morning. It was a difficult decision, but I chose to stay home and try to rest. Lightning thoughts pierced my mind, and my worries thundered so loudly in my head, I couldn't sleep.

I called a friend at four a.m. after David had left for the hospital. I sobbed, "My whole family is falling apart. Jake's got double-pneumonia. Andrew's going to the hospital, and they're going to admit him. He's got pneumonia. I'm going in for an ultrasound in the morning. I can hardly breathe and I'm sure I've got pneumonia too." Once again, I fell apart over the phone. My friend came right over and stayed with me until I had to leave for the doctor. I went to the doctor with my mom and sure enough, I had double-pneumonia. They also discovered that my baby was in the breech position. I was only two weeks from my due date. Andrew was hospitalized so that they could keep a close watch on him.

I had double pneumonia. Jake had double pneumonia. The baby was breech and we had to move the next day. This thunderstorm had turned into a full blown hurricane and I couldn't wait to find a little calm in the eye of it. My husband worked for a large hotel chain and they offered David and I a free room, to get away and relax. They knew about Andrew and that I was sick and they wanted to do something for us. David and I were supposed to meet there later that night. I was to help people pack us up at the apartment and he was going to stay at the hospital with Andrew all day. I couldn't be there because I was so sick. I rested that day and people came from our church and family and I directed them in what I wanted done and where I wanted things to go. Things seemed to be getting better, but the storm wasn't over yet.

My friend, Jeanne acted as my personal aide that day. She drove over to the hotel with me and we waited for David. Another friend, Debbie Murphy, stayed at the hospital with Andrew that night. She became close to him and to us and eventually we called her our "angel." She was truly a godsend. She helped me in more ways than I could ever recount or remember. I don't know what it would have been like if it wasn't for people like Debbie and others during that year. I don't think I would have made it. They were my strings to Jesus, because in my exhaustion and anger, I had cut off all ties to Him. They were the threads I was dangling on. I credit all of them for supporting me in very personal and practical ways.

When Jeanne and I reached our room, the hotel manager had started a fire in the fireplace for us. After he left, the flue broke or jammed and the fire began raging. Smoke started billowing into the hotel room. As the room became black with smoke, we raced around grabbing our luggage. We couldn't see in the darkness, because there was so much black smoke. The wall by the fireplace was completely black. Jeanne and I got out of there as fast as we could and there we were, standing out in the freezing January weather. We had no coats on, smoke was pouring out of our hotel room, and we waited for the hotel manager to come. Smoke alarms were blaring. It was chaotic, nothing like the calm I had hoped for, even for one night.

Our room was severely damaged because of the smoke, and we were upset and coughing. They gave us another room, and got us settled in. They apologized to us and I could tell they felt very badly, because they had known a little bit about our situation, and that I was very ill. It was just one more thing on top of it all. Finally, David arrived and we got settled for the night. I lay there questioning this bizarre chain of events wondering if it had a spiritual basis. Finally, only the distant rumbling of my sleepy thoughts could be heard as that storm retreated into the night.

The next day, the sun was shining. David and I left the hotel to visit Jake and to hang out with him for awhile. He was doing much better. The evening before he had been very uncomfortable, but he had improved significantly during the night. We stopped and picked up some things that we needed and came to our new house. It was about two o'clock in the afternoon when we arrived and during that whole day, family and friends had been moving us in. We started for the door, and about ten people walked past me in the driveway saying, "Bye, Leanne, Bye! Enjoy your new home." I didn't know any of them. I smiled at them and said, "Thanks" and I walked into the house.

Pictures were hung on the walls, people were sitting around the dining room table eating sloppy joes, and furniture was where it was supposed to be. I just kind of wandered through the house in awe. The kitchen was put in order, and the bathrooms. I walked upstairs and my bedroom had beautiful floral arrangements placed here and there.

My friend Elizabeth, the very first person I had called and told about Andrew's suspicious mass, was standing there putting some finishing touches in my room. Every room was adorable. I looked at her and she said, "Lay down. Don't do anything and just rest. Just lay down." And I did. I laid down and I cried, because I was so thankful that we finally had a home. We didn't know that we would eventually own the home, but it was enough that we had a home with enough room for our family, and that the move was over and done with. I was so relieved.

Our friends and family did everything they could so that we could just focus on Andrew. They really pulled together for us. Every year on January 10th, the day that we moved in, we've celebrated having our own home. We light candles and we buy some special sparkling juice. We praise the Lord for what He has given us, and we thank Him for the family and friends that supported us in the past and continue to support us as a family. We do it, not only to remind ourselves of how we began in this home, but how people supported us. We feel it's important to never forget that.

6

The Rigorous Routine of Treatments: How it controlled our lives

Late in January of 1994, we were getting ready to start Andrew's second round of chemo, and I was getting ready to deliver the new baby, Luke. Now that we were moved in, we had to focus on getting his breech posture turned around. We scheduled an external inversion. After sedating me, two doctors got on either side of me and they manipulated my swollen abdomen in order to turn the baby around. It hurt for a few minutes and then when it was done we hoped he would stay that way.

That night we had a prayer meeting at our house. During the meeting my friends prayed and laid their hands on me according to James 5:14, which says, "Is any one of you sick? He should call the elders of the church to pray over him and anoint him with oil in the name of the Lord." Then we prayed over every room in the house and also over Andrew. As we prayed and laid our hands on Andrew, he fell asleep. For me, Andrew's peacefulness was evidence of God's presence with us through what was only the very beginning of our extensive trials with him.

We started the second round of chemo in January of 1994. We had to time it along with the baby's arrival. Typically, Andrew had a couple of days that he would feel good and then he would get sick. So that it would be more convenient for us, I went into the hospital and they induced labor. That way, we wouldn't all of a sudden be delivering a baby when Andrew might be hospitalized because of low blood cell counts. Since the chemotherapy kills the cancer cells as well as healthy cells, the body's ability to fight disease or infection is weakened. When Andrew had very low blood cell counts, he was susceptible to disease, and we didn't want him to be sick when the baby came if we could help it.

My sister came to help at the end of January. That really saved me, because she did everything. A mother herself, she thought every thought I did and then she did it. She was one step ahead of me all the time as far as getting the meals and cleaning the house and watching the kids. She stayed up with Luke at night so that I could get some sleep and I remember feeling scared when she left, because I knew I was on my own with five children. But, like a baby eagle, I needed to be thrown out of the nest and learn to fly on my own. And I did. I didn't nurse Luke very long, maybe about two months. I couldn't focus on that because I was so involved with Andrew's care.

In February, Andrew had his treatment and as mentioned earlier, he was hospitalized three to three-and-a-half weeks out of every month. We spent a lot of time away from our children. Our prayers for them were very desperate during those times. I remember a friend reminding us that others were helping us in the Lord's name and if one of them was putting our children to bed it was like Jesus, himself was putting them to bed. That gave me a lot of comfort, because it was so hard to be separated from our family all the time. It was frustrating to be tossed about here and there and not have any control. I had absolutely no control over what I wanted, or the choices I wanted to make. People would call to talk and mention some great movie they'd just seen and David and I would be oblivious.

We had almost forgotten there was an outside world. The hospital was our world now. It's like a whole other planet. Anyone that's been in the hospital long term will say that it's like being in another world, a whole different environment. In the outside world where you are a "civilian", you can do what you please, but inside the hospital a controlled environment exists. You have very limited choices of what you can and can't do. It's very difficult to be in that atmosphere on a long term basis. Some people might be comforted by it, but I felt restricted and I didn't like it. I guess it went against the grain of my controlling nature, which I consider a weakness in myself, but there were times when I could feel God's grace help me to overcome it.

In March of 1993 they wanted to do a bone marrow harvest in Los Angeles. Our trip to California was overwhelming. Luke was six weeks old and I was nursing him, so we brought him along. We left Minneapolis on March 14th for Los Angeles and we stayed in Marina del Rey. We went into LA Kids where Andrew had two days of tests and the third day they did a bone marrow harvest. It was a scary time for David and I. We didn't know anyone in California. We didn't know how to get where we were going. It was shortly after the riots of 1992, and it was an unpredictable time out there. We were grateful that we could stay out in Marina del Rey because it was near the coast and calmer there.

After some pre-op tests at the hospital, we visited the Santa Monica pier to get some fresh air. We were struck by the numbers of people who were homeless and at first, we felt a bit fearful, yet we were strangely comforted by their presence. It was a reminder that there were others enduring hardships. We were not alone. Andrew did pretty well that day. I have a picture of he and I on that pier. His hair was thinning and scraggly. We bided our time until the bone marrow harvest which was scheduled for the next morning.

The procedure was excruciating for Andrew. They took out bone marrow from the base of his neck and lower back. It was cleaned up to make sure there was no cancer in it and then frozen. I wonder where it is now and if it is still frozen somewhere. I don't know what they do with it if it's not used. We went back to the hotel and poor little Andrew couldn't even move. He couldn't even turn his head he was in so much pain. He was just 22 months old then.

We returned home and did another round of chemo and again, we were in and out of the hospital. Andrew's blood counts would go down and he would get an infection. By then he was completely bald. We adjusted to the routine, but it was strenuous one. I don't remember much about that time. I certainly didn't have many opportunities to reflect on what was happening. I just had to follow the routine because it meant life or death for Andrew.

Every month brought new challenges and new illnesses and a new degree of Andrew's condition. His health was our main focus and anything else was just a luxury. If I wasn't on my way to the hospital, that was a luxury. If I could be in the grocery store, that was a luxury. Those things represented some sort of normalcy. If I could sleep in my own bed, if I could wash my clothes, those were luxuries. The disease controlled my life to the point where I appreciated things so much more. I try to remember that, because so quickly I can revert back to taking these simple everyday things for granted.

In May Andrew underwent five days of radiation treatments. The room was intimidating at first. With its huge, two-foot thick steel door, it looked like something from a James Bond movie. Inside, the walls were painted with murals for the patients to look at. Andrew was at an age where it was real touchy. He couldn't move. If he moved, they might radiate the wrong part of him, and could really damage something. I was told that if Andrew moved during that first treatment, they would sedate him that day and for the rest of the treatments, so I was very anxious. I did not want him to be sedated. Fortunately, the first day worked out great. They turned on "Barney" so Andrew could watch him. That was fun for Andrew and it really helped divert his attention and relieve his anxiety.

The radiation didn't take very long at all. It was just a zzzip-zap. I could go into another room and watch him on the monitor. I remember when I heard the machine click on I got such an eerie feeling. I wondered, "What am I doing to my child?" I hated those days because I never knew if I was doing the right thing. One wrong move could cause permanent damage. I wanted so much to run and take him off that table and protect him.

April, May, June, July, all of those months were filled with chemotherapy and weeks in the hospital. As a result of the chemotherapy, Andrew had marble-sized sores that began in his mouth, went down his esophagus and into his stomach, through his intestinal wall and into his rectum. He bled internally from them and there was blood in his stool. Also, he would vomit after the radiation treatments. He had been through so much by this time, it was hard to imagine him withstanding anymore.

7

Angry at God:Cancer takes an emotional toll

       I hesitated to include this episode in the book because it seems so self-centered. Then I was reminded that parents would be my most likely readers and I decided it would be important to include it for their sake. Battling cancer in a child not only drains a family physically and financially, but also emotionally. I include this story for those who will relate to what I went through so you will know that you are not alone. You'll probably find that you are coping much better than I did!

       In June, David left for his first Promisekeepers Convention in Denver, CO. Although we both wanted him to go, I had a very hard time emotionally. My spiritual health had deteriorated and I was very angry. I hated God and I felt like his puppet. Every time I talked to someone, I told them how I was God's puppet. I felt He was manipulating me and I was getting tired of it. One day, during David's absence, all I wanted to do was mow the lawn. All the kids were either satisfied, napping, or playing in the little plastic pool on the deck so I thought I'd give it a try. It was my only chance to get it done. I figured I had about 25-30 minutes to do it. I wanted to do something normal; something that would stay done for awhile.

       The lawnmower wouldn't start. I kept trying anyway. I pulled the cord back so many times that my fingers started bleeding because I had torn away the skin. I was not just angry and determined but out of my head with rage. I kept trying over and over. I refused to pray for God's help. I had

had so many struggles in my short life and was in the midst of a dealing with terminal cancer in one of my children. I thought I deserved to have the lawnmower start for me. I started screaming and swearing at the top of my lungs. I told God, "No way, You're treating me like I'm your puppet and you control me and I'm sick of it! What are you trying to do? I'm trying to change. All I want is to start this lawnmower and I'm not going to ask you for help." I pushed the lawnmower against a little woodshed next to our house and I rammed it into the trees and hit it against a tree a couple of times. I picked it up and dropped it a couple of times. The last thing I did was to pick it up above my head and drop it onto the ground!

I walked away swearing at God and telling him again that I wasn't going to ask him for help. It was a huge turning point, a beginning of my rebellion against God that lasted for a month or so. I was so angry that every aspect of our lives was totally and completely under the control of the disease and our exhaustive treatment program. I had no options. I had no choices. I couldn't get up in the morning and plan my day. We couldn't spontaneously head out for the beach that summer. The day was already completely planned out and we had to follow the plan because it meant life or death. I hated it. I was tired of it. For me, just wanting to start the lawnmower seemed like such a simple thing and I felt like God wouldn't even allow me to do that.

That whole summer of 1993 was a storm of emotion for me. I was rebellious and turning away from God. I started smoking. I started drinking. Not heavily, but whenever I could get out with a friend and go to a bar I would. I tried to get a cigarette whenever I could. I'd take off and go to the store and stop at the park on the way home and sit and smoke a cigarette. I started doing things that were typical of my old character and definitely not good for me, or those around me. I was too harsh with my kids. That same weekend, I was planning to go to my ten-year class reunion just a few miles away and our basement flooded. We don't know why it happened, but it destroyed all the carpet in our basement.

Our tenant downstairs was acting very strange toward me about the carpet and arguing with me. I didn't realize at the time that she was struggling with manic-depression and the problem with the carpet was magnified for her. Andrew was sick and I was trying to deal with his pumps and medications, along with getting ready for my reunion. David was still away at the Promisekeepers Convention. I began yelling at my kids and I knew I was close to losing control, so I sent them to their rooms so I could be alone to get a grip on myself and prepare to go out.

I climbed into the shower and I was immediately overwhelmed with horrid thoughts racing through my mind. I felt that at that moment I was being attacked spiritually. Satan's schemes were getting the best of me and I knew I had to get away from the house and the children. I threw on my robe and ran to my bedroom where I called my friend Michelle and said, "Michelle, you need to get down here right now. I'm really scared. I need to leave. I need to leave my kids for awhile. I'm falling apart and I'm just losing it. You need to come." She said, "I'll be there as fast as I can." While she was on her way, I packed a week's worth of food and clothes in the van. I wanted to get them in the van before she got there, so she wouldn't know that I didn't plan on coming back for weeks. I packed everything I could. I took as much money as I could, and the whole time, the kids stayed in their room. I didn't trust myself. As Michelle walked in the door, I walked out. I didn't even say anything to her. I got in the van and the first thing I did was stop and buy a pack of cigarettes. I hadn't smoked for six years and all of a sudden I was smoking a lot.

I drove all over the Minneapolis-St.Paul Metro area, and even through some small towns on the outskirts. I wanted to find a motel where I could stay because I didn't plan on going back, but I couldn't figure out how to do it without someone finding me. I didn't want anyone to track me down. I needed to find a place to go and get my head straight. All the while I was smoking cigarettes one after another. I was so sick with them that I started to vomit and my head started to pound. I knew I was in trouble then. I leaned over with my chest on the steering wheel. I prayed, "God, lead me somewhere safe."

The next thing I remember was pulling into my friend, Jeanne's driveway. She was there, and when she saw me, she realized I was in trouble. I told her I was at the end of my rope and I was going to leave my family. I couldn't take it anymore. I needed a place to rest because I didn't feel good.

I was so sick. She was leaving for work so she offered me her bed. She tucked me in, put water by the nightstand and told me to use anything I needed. It was only 6:30 p.m. but I fell right to sleep and woke up about four hours later. I went downstairs and saw a note from Jeanne telling me to make myself at home. She wrote that she had called her sister to let her know I was there and that I was not doing well. Her sister might check on me, or if I needed to call someone that was close, she was only about five minutes away. Jeanne encouraged me in her note not to go home but to stay and spend the night. I turned her note over and wrote, "Guilt is making me go back home. The guilt of leaving my children, and though I don't want to go back and know it isn't healthy, I can't live with this guilt." The guilt was more powerful than anything that could make me stay. When I arrived at home, Michelle was surprised to see me. I asked her to leave and I climbed into bed. I don't know how I started the next day. I don't remember how it began. I was really shaken up and felt I couldn't trust myself. I'd had a heck of a week. I spent the day getting the carpet out of the basement.

When David and his friend pulled in from their trip, David did the typical thing, whenever someone comes home from an exciting trip. He began telling me all about it. I barely heard him, I just looked at him. I wanted him to hold me, and I wanted to collapse in his arms and have him protect me and take care of me. He had no concept of what had gone on that weekend. It wasn't until later when he learned of the rough weekend I had, that he became very concerned and realized we were falling apart because of all this stress. He became stronger for my sake which helped get us through the rest of that summer.

Nevertheless, our marriage was really tense. We were handling the stress in different ways, and we weren't communicating to each other. I bugged him, he bugged me. He couldn't do anything right. I couldn't do anything right. I felt like I was pulling the whole load around the house and he was doing nothing. That is how David responds to stress. Although he is still feeling the frustration and the helplessness, he sort of shuts down, which is exactly opposite of me. I respond to stress by organizing and working and then resenting it. So we were fighting.

On one particular night, I don't remember why we were fighting, but I do remember Andrew's counts were bottoming out and he was sick. We were both exhausted, folding laundry, and we weren't communicating about something. I remember thinking, "I'm going to have to go to the hospital tonight. I'll call them and tell them he's vomiting, has a fever, junky cough, and blood in his stool, and they're going to tell me to bring him in." I just wanted to stay home. It's so much work to go into the hospital. As I held five-month old Luke, I told David how exhausted I was, and he was falling asleep on the couch. We fought about who was the most tired and who should go to the hospital. I really wanted him to go. He was saying that he had to go to work. I yelled, "#$!*@ work! I'm falling apart! Who cares about work?!" Well, we needed the money because we were falling apart financially, too. It was a terrible fight and we weren't getting anywhere with it.

He fell asleep on the couch while I went to make the phone call to the hospital. They told me to bring him in immediately. I yelled at David and he didn't even wake up. I started packing up and decided I would leave and I wasn't even going to talk to him. I wasn't going to tell him what was going on. I packed up the double stroller, all of Luke's needs and Andrew's needs, because I figured we would be there for a day or more. I put the kids in the car and as I was driving down the interstate, Andrew threw up. My mind raced back to the time when Jake couldn't breathe and I was rushing him to the emergency room. I had my flashers on going 85 mph through downtown Minneapolis. I was going to plow down anyone in my way because Jake wasn't breathing. (I could have easily pulled over and bagged him.) I knew I couldn't do anything for Andrew and he would have to wait until we got to the hospital. He had to just sit there with vomit on him.

I got to the ramp into the hospital. It was after midnight in a scary part of town. I was uncomfortable being there alone. I parked at the top of the ramp. The door to the hospital is situated in the middle of the ramp at the bottom. I got the stroller out and put Luke in it. I thought I had pushed down the brake. I was going to carry Andrew because he was so sick and so sad, but first I had to clean him up. Luke was in the stroller, along with the diaper bag and everything else. Andrew said something to tell me that he had to throw up. I held him away from me because I had only the clothes on my back with me. He vomited projectilely and thankfully, he missed me. I'm not sure if I bumped the stroller or what, but the next thing I knew, the stoller was rolling down the incline with Luke in it. Andrew was screaming and throwing up at the same time. I tried to hold him away from me as I ran after the stroller. When Andrew finished throwing up, I held him close to me so I could run faster to catch the stroller. It was picking up speed as it went down the slope.

Andrew said he had to throw up again. Running as fast as I could to catch the stroller, I held Andrew out away from me again. We were about midway down the ramp and I was still 10-15 feet away from the stroller. The stoller started to slow down, turn and head for a   parked car. Andrew finished vomiting again, and again, I held him close and ran after Luke. I had managed to keep my only outfit clean so far. Then Andrew threw up again, all down my back. He pushed himself away from the mess and threw up all down the front of me. Simultaneously, the stroller hit the parked car and Luke started screaming. Andrew was screaming and I was swearing like you would not believe.

We walked in to the hospital and the nurses met us with wide eyes. Luke had calmed down, but Andrew was still upset. I called home to tell David I needed him to come, because I couldn't do this alone. I was exhausted and I needed some support. The answering machine picked up and I screamed into the phone trying to wake him up. I couldn't get a hold of him and I was filled with resentment. It took me and the kids some time to get settled in. It was probably 3-4 a.m. before I calmed down and Andrew and I were cleaned up and showered. I couldn't take care of myself right away. I had to let them know what was going on with him and be there for him. Meanwhile, Luke was waking up and wanting to be fed. It was an awful, exhausting night.

The next day I still had Luke with me. David came after work so I could go home that night and David stayed. I came back the night after that with Luke and it was the worst experience. Luke would scream and fuss and I would finally get him to sleep and then Andrew would scream and fuss. I maybe slept for 20 minutes that night between dealing with the nurses and Luke and Andrew. I remember calling David at three in the morning and swearing over the phone. I couldn't get a hold of him. The phone upstairs was probably shut off and I got the answering machine. I was yelling into the machine, hoping that he would hear it and come down to listen to it. I said, "If you don't get up right now and come down here, I'm going to divorce you. I can't take this, I need sleep. I hate you!!!" The physical, emotional and spiritual exhaustion had taken its toll on me, my marriage and my family.

8

A Lesson From God

I didn't realize how precarious Andrew's condition was at that time. I stayed in that hospital room with him for four straight days, I thought about God and how I had watched Andrew suffer through so much pain. I had been a Christian for a few years, but the truth of John 3:16 reached into my heart for the first time that week. God gave his only begotten Son so that if we believe, we can come to know Him. We can be spared the punishment we deserve and have everlasting life.

I was sitting there holding Andrew and rocking him as I had been doing for the previous three days, and I had a daydream. In my dream, a crowd of people came in and grabbed Andrew out of my arms. They took him through some double glass doors. The people were beating him and whipping him. It all happened in slow motion. I was trying to get through the door to rescue Andrew. He was screaming and reaching for the safety of my arms. It took all the strength I had to get to Andrew. When I finally reached him and held him in my protective arms, the mob of people disappeared. Andrew was suddenly peaceful once again. Although my heart was still racing from the experience, I was comforted by the fact that I was able to save Andrew. I sat down in the hospital chair stroking Andrew's face, lulling him to sleep, when suddenly I realized Jesus was standing before us. I saw the look of compassion on his face and I knew that his heart ached for us and what we were going through. I felt that he wanted me to know that everything would be OK. While he stood there, the same mob of people that attacked Andrew rushed in and seized Jesus. They dragged him out through the corridor and began beating him, like they had done to

Andrew. That's when it struck me that God had the power to
rescue Jesus and he didn't. He didn't stop Jesus' suffering and
whippings and beatings and torture and crucifixion, because
He loved *me* so much. He had to allow Jesus to endure those
things so there would be sufficient payment for my sin. It was
such a powerful illustration. God broke through to my heart
that day. I had been pretty distant and focused only on what
we were doing with Andrew. I believed then, to my very core,
that God loved me. He loved me and he let his Son die for
me. If someone was hurting my child, I could intervene and
rescue him. God had even more power to do that for his son
than I ever will have, and he didn't! The truth of God's love
had finally reached deep into my heart.

9

Yellow Flowers and a White Casket: Planning Andrew's funeral

Towards the end of the chemotherapy treatments I realized that our options for Andrew were running out. I became obsessed with planning his funeral in my mind. I knew who would sing and who would speak. The colors would be yellow and white. Yellow is Andrew's favorite color, so there would be yellow and white flowers everywhere and I wanted to try to have that be the only colors. I knew it would be almost impossible, but David and I would request that anyone who wanted to send flowers, have them be yellow and white because it would really mean something to us.

His funeral was going to be open-casket and we were going to sing a couple of praise songs. A bunch of close friends and relatives would gather around his casket, just before we closed it. I told my mom and a couple of good friends about my plans because I knew that we would be in the hospital, and that we would be under a lot of stress. We didn't want anyone making those decisions for us. We were very specific about what we wanted. The yellow and white flowers and an open casket.

The casket would be white. Andrew would have on his little denim hat that he wore all the time. I will always save that hat because it has a lot of special memories. Andrew was adorable in it. It didn't matter that he was bald because he had his little hat. To this day, Andrew loves to wear hats. He would be dressed in his little denim shirt and jeans and look like a little rugged guy in a beautiful white casket covered with yellow flowers.

We made sure that we had all the songs picked out. There was a funeral home really close to our church and we were going to go there and have the wake. At the visitation we would display pictures of Andrew. My sister, Lynn, was going to make a collage of pictures and have captions. I imagined us working on it the night before and I thought it would have been healthy for David and I to look over pictures.

My sister, Lisa, was going to read scriptures we had picked out. The very first verse that jumped out at David and I when Jake was born was John 9:1-3. "As he went along, he saw a man blind from birth. His disciples asked him, 'Rabbi, who sinned, this man or his parents, that he was born blind?' 'Neither this man nor his parents sinned,' said Jesus, 'but this happened so that the work of God might be displayed in his life.'" Shortly after Jake finally got stable and we were able to relax a little, Andrew was diagnosed and as a parent, the first thing I thought was, "What am I doing wrong, God? What did I do? Why are you punishing me?" I questioned God like that for a long time. I didn't fully understand the God I was putting my faith and trust in for my salvation. That to me, is the key, to faith. If we don't understand the God we put our faith and trust in, how can we surrender our lives to Him? How can we possibly trust and put faith in a God that we don't know, much less, a God that we have assumptions or misconstrued ideas about. It helped us to remember that verse, because we didn't blame ourselves for Andrew's illness and we held on however feebly at times, to the hope that God's work would be displayed somehow in Andrew's life, or possibly in his death.

My sister would also talk about another verse in depth and the life application of it. It was Philippians 3:10, "I want to know Christ, and the power of his resurrection and the fellowship of sharing in his sufferings, becoming like him in his death." She was going to illustrate how Andrew had fulfilled that verse. He shared in the fellowship of Christ's sufferings here on earth by enduring torturing physical pain. If he had died of cancer, he would have known Christ intimately at that moment as well as the glorious power of his resurrection as he stood alive with him in Heaven. And like Jesus in his death, Andrew was innocent, a sort of sacrifice for the sin in this world. Jesus' sacrifice on the Cross was sufficient for our sin, but Andrew's death would not have been sufficient, for cancer cannot be satisfied. It keeps demanding sacrifices, and all of us are forced to give somehow, with our own life, or the life of a loved one.

At the funeral, Pastor Mark would share an evangelistic message of hope to the people that have not heard the gospel and then David and I would speak. We viewed the funeral as a great big Thank You card. A thank you to God for allowing us to spend time with Andrew. Even though the years were short, we would thank God for the opportunity to be blessed by the experience of loving him.

We wanted to use the opportunity to thank everyone for things they did for us. We would thank the people who contributed money, who cleaned our house, who put contact paper on the kitchen cupboards when we moved in. We'd thank all the people who not only moved us, but cleaned the apartment that we moved out of, the house that we moved into, and unpacked all of our things. It took a lot of stress off our entire family. Half the time, we didn't know who did things. We knew who was in charge of delegating things, but had no idea that it was all going on. We would thank the people that faithfully brought meals to the hospitals for weeks. We'd thank the people that watched our kids and who did special things for the other kids when we couldn't be there to do it.

We wanted to thank the people who gave parking money at the hospital. It's so expensive, especially when you are going there two or three times a day. Thank you to the people who would come and wash our laundry, or drop off something we needed. Thank you to the people who made phone calls for us. The church had a group of people come and clean the house twice a week or once every Saturday. Thanks to those who cleaned out the fridge, cleaned out our cars, or took the van in to be worked on. Some people even videotaped our kids and then brought the tape up to us at the hospital so we could see them. Thank you to the people who bought us books of encouragement. Thank you to the people who prayed. Thank you to Sue Bird who brought me cards with verses that I still carry with me today.

Out of the compassion of their hearts people rallied together and donated a large sum of money. Our pastors told them that we were in need and I think the congregation was horrified at our situation with Andrew, because they had seen Jake's struggle for life also. With the money that was donated, we were able to put a down payment on our house and even buy another used vehicle so David had a car to go to work and I had a car to go to the hospital. David and I were going to try our best at the funeral to thank everyone and bring up everything we could remember. Even the little things which are the most important during hard times.

10

Our last chance:Another attempt at removing the tumor

Towards the end of July we were winding up conventional treatment with Andrew's last round of chemo. It was something we were looking forward to, but we knew afterwards, if we hadn't destroyed the tumor, we were in a lot of trouble. We entered the latter part of the summer with great apprehension because we knew life and death decisions were going to have to be made.

By now, Andrew was completely bald. He was twenty-six months old and weighed only 24 lbs. His blood counts were really low and he was very vulnerable to common illnesses. His diet was still very poor and he was understandably whiney and clingy.

August 2, 1993 was Andrew's last day of chemotherapy. We spent the rest of August in the hospital. They sent us home and decided that they would give Andrew a little time to recuperate from that last round of chemo and then we would talk about trying again to remove the tumor surgically. They didn't feel he would be a good candidate for a bone marrow transplant unless the tumor was removed. Our doctors decided to consult a world famous doctor from Europe, who was well-known for removing tumors from difficult places.

When the time came for surgery, we did all the pre-operative procedures down in Rochester, Minnesota at the Mayo Clinic for about a week. I was early in my pregnancy with my sixth child, Lauren. The day of the surgery I was sick. At 7 a.m. I was holding Andrew, waiting for him to be taken into the operating room. My dad and my sister came to be with us. David's parents came, too. Some friends from church showed their support by being there and we all stood there together waiting. It was a very emotional time. It's hard to describe the feeling. Once again, as I was holding my child, preparing to hand him over to a surgeon I felt the familiar, ugly fear. Andrew was adorable, smiling, cuddly and alive and I knew that I would not get him back like that. I'd gone through the same experience several times with Jake and now several times with Andrew, but I never got used to it. It's an incredible experience. I put a child in someone's hands, and they make the judgment calls. It's an utterly helpless position and one must trust completely, whatever the outcome.

We knew that this surgery was our last chance. They had warned us that there was only a 2% chance that Andrew would come out of the surgery alive with the tumor successfully removed. And if he lived through it but they were unable to remove the tumor, we understood that it meant Andrew's treatment would be over and we would have to take him home to die. A bone marrow transplant was Plan B, but it was futile to attempt unless they could remove the tumor. If that didn't happen, there was nothing more for us to do. Andrew's life was suspended on a thin shred of hope, yet we clung to it with all our might. He went into the operating room that day and the surgery team opened him up to prepare him for the famous surgeon. Later, the team recounted to us what happened in the operating room. The doctor had come in, taken one look at where the tumor was, threw up his hands and said, "No way. I am not touching this child." He also told them he felt that any attempt to remove the tumor would take Andrew's life. And then he walked out! The rest of them stood there dumbfounded, but they decided to attempt to remove what they could, and would stop if it got too dangerous. The surgery team emerged from the operating room and told us they had been unsuccessful and had only removed about 15% of his tumor. They told us openly that they removed areas of the tumor in such a way as to ease the pain for Andrew while he was dying.

We were crushed. We felt an urgent desire to get to Andrew, to cherish him, spend time with him, and cuddle him close to us. We hoped he would recover quickly so that we could leave the hospital and go home as soon as possible.

Now that a cure for Andrew was so far out of our reach, our position shifted to one of protection for him. We just wanted out of that hospital.

A friend of ours stayed down in Rochester with us. She was going to sleep right next to Andrew that night so David and I could go and sleep in a lounge and get some rest. We hadn't slept much at all that week, because we were doing pre-op tests with Andrew. We were just exhausted. Just before we were to leave Andrew for the night a young oncologist came in. We began asking her what our options were. We asked her about experimental chemo, because we had heard about it in different conversations with doctors. It would be mentioned, but was never described in detail to us. She crossed her arms over her chest very abruptly and she said, "Face it. Your son is going to die from this." We had been grasping at straws, so much so that it became irritating to those trying to help us. I believe that in her mind those words were intended to help us realize that there was nothing more for us and possibly she felt she needed to be that frank so we could accept it. Maybe it was the right thing for her to say, because at that point we became truly desperate and turned our search wholly toward God.

We prayed a lot for Andrew to have a good recovery, and asked others to pray also. He did recover amazingly quickly and we went home. We were home in a matter of three days after his surgery. As I walked in the door, my little brown suitcase still in hand, the phone was ringing. It was the Minneapolis Childrens' Hospice Program. A very gracious woman said, "I understand you have a dying child in your home. We understand Andrew is dying of cancer and we would like to know if you would like us to come out to set up and get familiar with Andrew, and your family and see how we could best assist in the death of your child." I was stunned, but I managed to say, "You know, not at this point. We just got home. We are a little overwhelmed, call me back in a couple of days." And I hung up. I remember standing there and tears started rolling down my face, because *they* were all done. They were all showing us how they had been communicating behind the scenes. In their human estimation, the next phase for this family was to assist or support in the death of this child. It was a terrible moment for both David and I, yet we had five children running around our feet and we had to take care of the domestic duties and maintenance involved with the family. We busied ourselves with that until later that night.

11

God Makes a Way

As we sat down at about 11:00 p.m. that night, and began to ponder our few options, we started to pray. We were completely humbled and asked for God's mercy. In painful surrender we cried out to our Father for help. We were totally and completely dependent upon Him. We asked God to show us another way. We asked Him to show us how to help Andrew and to heal him. We asked him to forgive us for seeking just man's wisdom in healing Andrew's cancer. That's when the two books, *A Cancer Battle Plan* and *Prescription for Nutritional Healing* came into our lives.

A lady that I don't even know out in Oregon sent us *Prescription for Nutritional Healing*, because she thought we could benefit by reading it. She sent it home with her visiting daughter-in-law who knew me from our church. That book and what it taught me about cancer in a short amount of time changed the whole direction of our lives. The books were sitting on our countertop. I didn't even know they were there. Apparently somebody had dropped them off for us. It was a miracle that they happened to be there that night when we prayed. After we prayed, I immediately got up and walked over to the counter, picked up the book, turned to cancer and started reading. I said, "Oh my gosh!" I sat back down on the couch with David and I read and read. I said, "We've gotta try this. We've gotta do this!" David wholeheartedly agreed. Suddenly, we were given a new sense of hope. We discovered there was something constructive that we could do for the first time since Andrew was diagnosed. That was the most significant thing. The authors of these books were saying, "Try this", and "Do this." Throughout Andrew's traditional therapies no one suggested that there were things we could do for him at home. David and I were elated that there were proactive things that we could do. It made such a difference to us. When we were unaware of nutritional therapy we were trapped by the disease. Our ignorance had us backed into corner we couldn't escape. Our only hope was to try feebly to deal with the stress.

We called our friend Dr. Pete Wurdemann who is a chiropractor. He had been sharing tidbits of information throughout Andrew's course of conventional therapy, but we weren't open to it. We were now at the point where we were completely surrendered and open to learning about it. We called him and told him we wanted to try it. We asked him what the treatment entailed. He told us Andrew needed megadoses of vitamins, chiropractic care, and lots of fresh, organic carrot-apple juice. I asked him if he would help us. We had to go in the next day to talk to our oncologist about putting Andrew on experimental chemo, but we didn't feel very good about it. In fact, we had bad feelings about the idea. When we had asked her about it previously she told us that it would maybe prolong his life a month or two but his quality of life would be really poor. He would be in the hospital and he would be sick all the time.

We told Dr. Pete that we were going in the next morning at 9:00 a .m. and asked if he would come with us and support us, because we really didn't know what we were talking about. He said he would, and the next day he, Andrew, and David and I and went to our appointment. Our doctor had invited another oncologist from the University of Minnesota, who was heading up the experimental chemo program. She introduced him and he began to "sell" us on the idea of experimental chemo. When it became apparent to them that we had other plans for Andrew, and their program was not part of those plans, it turned into an awkward situation. Our oncologist abruptly left the room for a few minutes, while the other doctor listened to what we wanted to do, but of course, he was biased to what his option offered. Eventually, they became more and more frustrated because they weren't getting anywhere with us. They both left the room and had a conversation in which I assume they conceded that they were not going to convince us to take their route. My general feeling was that they were frustrated with us and perturbed by what we were pursuing.

Finally, they gave up and our oncologist came in and said, "I am biased to drug therapy. It's all I know, but I don't have any options for you. If you want to pursue this, I will support you in any way I can." That's when we said to her, "Great. We want you to place a G-tube into Andrew. We are familiar with the gastrostomy procedures because of our experience with Jake. We want to try it with Andrew because we need to get a lot of organic carrot-apple juice and lots of vitamins into him and we feel that this is the best way." We were dealing with a two-and-a-half year old who would be unable to swallow pills or take that amount orally even if they were crushed.

I think that our doctor was surprised at the boldness of our plan, yet also intrigued by it. She was supportive regarding the G-tube and we scheduled it immediately. It was in place within three days.

12

The Program

We started nutritional therapy in mid-to-late October of 1993. The first difference I noticed after beginning Andrew's nutritional therapy was *hope*. There was hope in our household. A new sense of hope; a fresh beginning. We held anticipation for the future now, along with the anxiety and fear that had become common in our everyday lives. Nutritional therapy made sense to us. We learned that in conventional therapy, we were actually destroying Andrew's immune system, and now we needed to build it up. We were willing to do whatever it took.

The next thing I realized was the awesome amount of responsibility that I had taken on. I was deluged with information, and I became mentally exhausted. At first, I didn't want to know why I was doing the things I was doing for Andrew. Dr. Pete and his wife Lisa, set up his protocol and gave us a list of things to do. They would try to give me some basic information on the reasons for doing them, but I just remember that initially, our task was to build up his immune system in order to help his body fight the disease. I was taught that the way to build up his immune system is through vitamins, minerals, protein and pure water. I could remember those simple things and when they said, "Here's betacarotene. It supports the liver, etc." I would say, "Don't tell me that. I'll learn that later. I'll do it until I'm comfortable with it and I'll learn more about it later." I was committed to giving Andrew nutritional therapy, but I couldn't absorb all the information so fast because I was so busy doing the hands-on work of the program.

The first physical thing I noticed with Andrew was his amount of elimination. When we started to give his body the good nutrients, they worked to cleanse his body and rid it of the toxins that had built up. We were hopeful this process would eliminate the cancer altogether. There was so much that sometimes Andrew would literally be laying in puddles of stool on my hardwood floor. Occasionally, the stool would have black chunks in it and I wondered if it was dried blood from internal bleeding, or if it was parts of the tumor. I never knew; I never took it in to be tested and, I didn't care. I just knew that it didn't look good and I was glad it was coming out of him. The stools were very foul-smelling. I knew that was a good sign, too. Dairy can make stools really foul-smelling, and it was like that. I knew that basic one-line concept that this elimination process was good. Basically, if it's really stinky and there is a lot of it, it's a good thing. The body is being cleansed of it.

I wanted to go in for tests after two weeks of treatment, but I couldn't because that would not have been enough time to see much of a change. Dr. Wurdemann encouraged us to wait until the first of the year which would make it a full ninety days before Andrew was tested.

In January of 1994 we scheduled a urine test and a blood test. Our doctor was amazed and told us that Andrew was gaining weight for the first time since he had been diagnosed in 1992. He had always maintained about 23-24 lbs., and at two-and-a-half years old he had finally reached 26lbs. Also, his blood and urine tests revealed that the cancer cells were decreasing in number. These great results reinforced our committment to nutrition and we continued Andrew's rigorous treatment.

It seemed like I was in the kitchen all day long preparing vitamins and juice for Andrew. I would take all the vitamin supplements and grind them in a coffee grinder. I would make fresh organic carrot-apple juice with a juicer. Andrew still used a bottle, so I would make two bottles of the juice. After I cleaned up the juicer, I would mix the vitamins with about five ounces of the juice. I would strain this to get the capsule parts from the vitamin E and betacarotene out, because that wouldn't go through the tube. I would let it soak, but not for too long, because I didn't want it to lose the live enzymes in the juice. Andrew would sit on the counter and I would put this juice and vitamin mixture into his tube.

When I finished the whole process, I would need to start all over again for noontime. I would set him to drinking his juice while I made lunch for the other kids and then began to prepare another round of vitamin-juice mixture for his G-tube. Then I'd clean up the kitchen once more. I would repeat the process again at suppertime, not to mention making meals for everyone else and learning what kind of meals we should be eating. In support of Andrew, we committed our whole family to a diet of 80% live foods, which is fresh, organic raw fruits and vegetables. The other 20% of our diet was whole grains like whole brown rice and whole wheat breads.

I was overwhelmed with the work and stretched to my limits continually. I had so much responsibility and for Andrew's sake I could not afford to neglect any part of his treatment. I was resentful because David could leave his work and come home. I couldn't, my work surrounded me constantly. Initially, he didn't learn how to prepare the juice and vitamins, because I did it all. I was angry that he didn't know what to do. He didn't know how much of the different supplements Andrew took. Eventually, he became more involved, but the bulk of responsibility was mine, because David was working during the day to support the family.

We all stayed at home more. Andrew's treatment limited our time to be out of the house, because I had to be around the juicer. We didn't go places as a family very much for about a year. We were certainly at the hospital and doctor's office a lot less. We went to a doctor appointment at three months and then again at six months. At the second appointment, our doctor came in with lab results and said, "It's a miracle! There are no cancer cells in Andrew's blood or urine, the tumor is soft and appears to be dormant." She declared Andrew "cancer free" after six months of nutritional therapy. Two appointments in six months was a major difference from spending three weeks out of every month living at the hospital.

We had been able to afford the nutritional program for about six months just by approaching people personally and asking for financial help. We didn't have a good system for managing the money and decided we needed a good system that would be more stable. The idea of setting up a nutrition fund came through prayer. We sat up until two in the morning one time praying with some friends of ours about what to do. Afterwards, someone mentioned the idea. We sent out a letter to our friends and family stating what we had learned about nutritional therapy, and the results we had achieved so far. Sadly, this form of healthcare is not covered by insurance, and we had to admit that we could not continue to provide Andrew with what he needed with our own resources. We believe that God led us to ask for help this way. We sent the letter out and found someone to manage the fund, so that it would not be another responsibility for us. Also, we thought it would be good ethically and would make people feel comfortable that we were not managing their money without some accountability. When we needed to buy something for Andrew's protocol, we would and the fund would pay us back. Sometimes we would get a blank check so we could go to the natural food co-op and purchase 50lbs of organic carrots and then bring the receipt back to the person who managed the fund. We got very positive responses from people we asked to support us. Everyone gave in some way or another and the fund continued for a couple of years.

13

Discovering the cause of our health problems

After one year of nutritional therapy the most significant benefit we noticed for Andrew was his exceptional quality of life compared to suffering through conventional medical therapy. He was running and laughing and having fun. His hair grew back and his eyes lit up. You could see the life in his eyes. There was no more vomiting. There were no more sores, and no more pain. He was eating well. He enjoyed the carrot-apple juice. There was nothing negative in Andrew's life at that point. I think the hardest thing for him was having to sit on the counter and wait for me to get the vitamin-juice mixture into him, so he could go off and play.

After two years his quality of life was much the same. He was ALIVE! He was experiencing the things that little children should experience. He was going to the beach and playing outside. He was swinging in the backyard and going for rides on the back of our bikes. We were able to hug and kiss him, and watch him play. For the first time since he was diagnosed, he was beginning to have a consistent quality of life.

In May of 1995, as part of researching more treatment for Andrew, I went and had a colonic done for myself with a naturopathic doctor. I told her our story and she was intrigued. She said she knew a doctor in New Hope that studied difficult cases like Andrew's. She talked to him and he was very impressed with what we were doing nutritionally for Andrew. He asked if we would travel down to Flagstaff, AZ to be studied at a conference of natural health doctors where they could ask us some questions and discuss Andrew's case. We were told that we might be able to find the cause of our childrens' health problems, and see if there was any different protocol they might suggest for Andrew. Financial help from our local food co-op, friends and family made the trip possible for us.

There were about 40-50 doctors present as we walked into a conference room. We were extremely intimidated. They had lap-top computers and books piled high on either side of them. We were seated in front of them all and they began asking very intense questions about our family's physical well-being, especially Andrew's. They asked about our emotional health and even asked Andrew some questions. The first session was about five hours long and the next day, we spent three hours answering questions.

Towards the end of the second day, the instructor, who had always been in the back of the room guiding the doctors' inquiries finally asked me, "Leanne, have you ever had problems with skin eruptions?" I thought, "Boy, that's an odd question, but I had had problems with acne." So I told him that after the birth of my first child, I had broken out with severe cystic acne. He asked me what I did about it and I told him I went to a dermatologist who put me on a drug called Accutane. What went on in that room after I said "Accutane" puzzled me. Some doctors put their faces in their hands. Some threw their pens up in the air and some even stood up and walked out of the room. A definite frustration and sadness filled the entire room.

As I sat there wondering what I had said, the instructor walked toward me to the front of the room. He looked down at me, put his hand on my shoulder and with tears in his eyes he said, "Leanne, I am so sorry for you." He turned around to the class and asked, "What do we know about the long-term side effects of Accutane?" I thought, "How strange, I've always heard of short-term side effects, but never long-term side effects."

That day I learned the long term side effects of Accutane. It distresses the central nervous system, it causes insomnia, **birth defects,** liver toxicity. It causes geno-toxicity, which means it can affect my children's children. It can cause pressure on the brain, urinary infections, gastro-intestinal infections, dizziness, seizures, **cancer**, a recurrence of acne, heart murmurs, eye damage, pains in the chest, legs and arms.

I had taken Accutane for about six months. A year and a half after I discontinued Accutane, I got pregnant with my second child, Jake. Jake is eight years old. He was born with a severe heart and stomach defect. He has a life-expectancy of his mid-to-late teens. He has had three open-heart surgeries. He has had a total of nine operations on his chest and his stomach. However, I would like to add that this has been Jake's best year yet healthwise. Typically, he gets double-pneumonia three to five times a year. This year he has been my healthiest child because we put him on a nutritional protocol.

My second child after taking Acutane is Aubree. She is six years old. Aubree has a mild heart defect which can be corrected by angioplasty. Andrew is my third child after Accutane. He is five and had terminal cancer. Next is Luke. He is three and he has gastrointestinal problems and urological problems. My fifth child after Accutane is Lauren. She is two years old. While I was pregnant with her I was pursuing a natural diet and food supplements, so I think that she has a fighting chance, yet I am apprehensive because Aubree and Andrew were not diagnosed until they were toddlers.

Since we've returned from Arizona, I have taken it upon myself to be tested by two different clinics. I never thought much about my health, I knew I had problems, but I was too overwhelmed and consumed with my two boys that were terminally ill. This is what I learned after being tested:

One doctor told me that my liver, adrenal glands and thyroid are severely stressed, and I have a pre-cancerous condition in my bladder. I was immune-suppressed. He said that my body was just on the edge of exploding into disease. It was then that I began a serious food supplement and detoxification program and I have seen positive results.

One quote from a doctor says, "Accutane is so toxic, it just doesn't seem worth the risk to put it on the market." To date, we know three doctors who are willing to testify that Accutane is the cause of the problems in four out of our six children, a naturopath, a chiropractor who is also a nutritionist, and a medical doctor. Also, the FDA didn't want Accutane on the market believing it was too risky, but the dermatology group fought for it because it had fast-acting results. One doctor also said, "Most drugs aren't tested for their long-term side effects. We typically see those side effects show up in the people that take the drug." One current example is the breast implants. We saw the long-term effects of those later on in the women who used them.

We left the conference in Flagstaff, AZ and began the six hour drive to Albuquerqe, New Mexico for the first leg of our trip home. We had borrowed a van equipped with a TV and VCR and we started a movie for the kids. David and I looked at each other again, like we had always done when we found out something incredible. We believed it made sense, but didn't know what to do next. We talked and I wondered aloud what I needed to do about my own health. I was relieved to learn that our problems were not just some fluke of nature, but there was a rational cause for our circumstances. It wasn't that God was bombarding us with trials because he was angry with us or that he wanted to refine our character. There was a real, material cause for our severe health problems. David and I were greatly comforted by this news and couldn't wait to tell others what we had learned at the conference.

My experience in Arizona renewed my passion for nutritional therapy. I was driven to share with others that there are options other than drug therapy. David and I told everyone we could, whenever we had the opportunity. We wanted others to benefit from what we had lived through. There are a few people around the country that we have been in contact with who are pursuing a course of nutritional therapy similar to Andrew's. There is one little boy with neuroblastoma in Rhode Island. His parents had a G-tube placed in him and his tumors are decreasing because of nutritional therapy. There is a little boy in Michigan that we know of who has followed Andrew's program and is also doing well.

Currently, Andrew's state of health is very stable. Medically, there are no cancer cells present in his blood or urine. He has not been to a doctor appointment for over a year. In the last conversation I had with a radiologist about Andrew's tumor, he stated that the tumor was soft and had not grown, but in fact was diminished in size and his assessment was that it was dormant. He added that there was no reason why Andrew shouldn't be expected to live as he is for 60-70 years.

Emotionally, Andrew faired very well throughout the whole ordeal. He understood that he had cancer and that it could kill him. He understands why he takes the supplements. He knows that they build up his immune system which fights the cancer. Every day, Andrew is given a small dish containing 40 supplements. At only five years of age, he can swallow them one at a time with water, although he likes to have someone sit with him while he does it.

The change in Andrew's quality of life has been dramatic. He spent the 4th of July this year, 1996, visiting his cousins in Ohio so my sister and I could get together to work on this book. Previously, trips that far from home were unfathomable. He is happy, and bubbly. He has a sweet disposition which he displays often. He's a very intelligent child and he started kindergarten this fall, right on schedule.

BOOK II
Key Points of Nutritional Therapy for Cancer

1

We are responsible: How our environment increases cancer risk

About halfway through our program we became aware of the many chemical culprits in our everyday environment and their impact on our health. Our immune systems can be depleted by pollution, chemical cleansers, poor water quality and poor diet. These factors reduce the body's abiltity to heal itself. We have seen a lot of positive changes being made, such as buildings becoming smoke-free, recycling programs, and the production of more all-natural products and generally, people are more health conscious today, but do they think much about what's in the water that comes from their tap? Do they wonder about the quality of the fresh fruits and vegetables they eat? How about the cleaners and disinfectants they use in their homes, do they ever question that they might be harmful? If you suffer from any disease, it may be time to closely examine your personal environment and see what you can do to make changes for your health's sake.

There are things we can control and things we can't control. We can't control being stuck in rush hour traffic and breathing in exhaust from other cars, but we can try to schedule errands and trips during times when there is less traffic. If we exercise outdoors, we can do it during the early morning hours when there is less exhaust in the air.

When it comes to inside our homes, we can change what we use for disinfectants and cleaners, as well as skin care products from chemically-based products to natural, biodegradeable, ph balanced products.

Switching to natural products is a significant way to make your home safer. When you use a soap to wash your skin or your child's skin, whether it's a natural product or not the skin absorbs it. Our skin breathes just like our lungs, and what we put on it, will be absorbed into our bodies. For Andrew's sake and our own, we changed everything in our home to natural products; cleaners, laundry soap, fabric softener, shampoo, etc. You would be amazed to add up the amounts of chemicals you probably keep and use in your very own home. You may even be very proud of your cleanliness, but you may be leaving a dangerous chemical residue wherever you clean. In our society today, there exists a heightened awareness toward our environment, but with a cancer patient in the family, you need to be more conscious of what you are using to clean that person's personal environment, including their clothes and their skin.

Access to pure water is vitally important. I met with a lady from a small town in Minnesota just south of where we live. She is very involved in her community. In that particular town, they believe that because of the poor water quality, five people have been diagnosed with brain tumors. That's frightening, and it's happening all over the country. We attend church in a town about 20 miles west of us, and there are twelve people in that congregation alone dealing with terminal cancer. What does that tell us about the water in that community? What has seeped into their ground water? We need to ask these questions and address the problem. It's such a big problem, and it's going to take a lot of time to make our community water supply safe for everyone. Meanwhile, as individual residents, we can take initiative and invest in a home water treatment system to help make our personal evironment as safe as possible. The Associated Press recently reported that water agencies are now required to make public yearly reports informing customers of the chemicals and bacteria that their tap water contains. Also, they must notify the public within 24 hours when a contaminant poses a significant risk.

Today, our food is depleted of nutrients before it even reaches us. We are suffocated by air pollution and poisoned with the water from our own kitchen taps. If you make these simple changes in your personal environment, you will never have to look back and wonder what disease you *didn't* get from the chemical products you formerly used. A look at your family's medical history might show that your grandparents had heart disease, diabetes, or cancer. If you change your diet and environment now, you can look forward to breaking these patterns of disease in you and your children. The question to ask yourself is, "What do I want out of life?" You could live to be 70-80 years old. That's a long time to be poisoning a body with chemicals and poor food. If you aren't willing to make positive changes and take responsibility for your environment and what you are ingesting, you may well end up living that long, but will most likely be weak, depressed and riddled with degenerative disease because of a weakened immune system.

It's important for the young people today to realize that they have this responsibility and there is constructive action they can take. They too, need to change their habits to deal with today's "in" diseases, such as AIDS, cancer, depression, chronic fatigue syndrome and acne, rather than popping a pill that could ultimately be detrimental to their health, longevity, and vitality. We all need to be willing to work for a healthy future by changing our personal living habits in the present. In the book *How To Get Well*, Paavo Airola, Ph.D. writes, "Cancer is a disease of civilization. It is the end result of health-destroying living and eating habits, which result in biochemical imbalance, and physical and chemical irritation of the tissues." Ultimately, it is our environment and our poor eating habits that have caused the epidemic of cancer in our country. It's time to take action to protect ourselves and our children from these elements.

2

A Weak Immune System:
The real cause of cancer

80-90% of all cancers are the result of things that we do to ourselves. In *A Cancer Battle Plan,* Dave and Anne Frahm quote Patrick Quillin, Ph.D. as stating, "New estimates say that 90% of all cancer is environmentally caused and hence, preventable. A conservative estimate states that 30-60% of all cancer is nutrition related. The U.S. has 50% more breast and colon cancer than any other areas of the world and much of this dubious distinction is caused by poor nutrition."

Every person has some amount of cancer cells in their body. And we have all been exposed to environmental and nutritional factors. When our immune system becomes weak, the cancer cells can mutate and become life-threatening. They start to reproduce and do not get the signal from the body that they have to stop. They begin to invade healthy tissue and organs or form hard masses, becoming cancerous tumors.

So, basically cancer is a symptom of your body's degeneration. In her book, *The Conquest of Cancer,* Dr. Virgina Livingston-Wheeler writes, "Cancer is a disease of the immune system, or more accurately a disease of a weak immune system. Your immunity must drop to a very low level before cancer can grow. When it drops to an extremely low level, the cancer cells start to spread. Your body has no defense against them and what small defense it has is not enough." I am convinced that nutritional therapy and natural healing for cancer treats the cause of the illness (a weak immune system) and not just the symptoms.

Poor nutrition and environmental factors are believed to be the two major causes of cancer. Securing a healthy immune system and maintaining that health is critical for the prevention and treatment of this disease. Your immune system builds healthy cells, and when your cells are healthy, they are able to fight infection or anything else that comes your way through your diet or environment. Degenerative diseases such as cancer, can be reversed through nutritional therapy. You cannot give up even if you are told by a doctor that cancer has spread throughout someone's entire body, and it's a hopeless situation. It's never a hopeless situation when dealing with a degenerative disease unless you choose to make it hopeless. This puts the responsibility on you to work feverishly to get you or your child's body back on track. You need to have a "do whatever it takes" mentality and as long as you understand the basics, you can get started right away.

Dr. Quinllan said 30-60% of all cancers are nutrition related. What if he is right? Doesn't it make sense to build up your body's immune system by eating foods that your body can use? It needs foods that are not loaded with chemical fertilizers and pesticides or cooked incorrectly, so that there is little nutritional value left in them. Organically grown, whole foods are your option. There are natural food stores out there, you just have to take a proactive stance and find them. Look in your local yellow-pages. There are stores and co-ops that are eager to help educate people so that they can have a more abundant life through eating right.

I learned that Andrew's immune system needed to be rebuilt. His cells needed proper vitamins, minerals and protein in order to become healthy enough to start fighting his disease from the inside-out. The basics to rebuilding your immune system are providing vitamins, minerals and protein through high quality food supplements, eating raw whole foods that are organically grown, and supporting the liver through a detoxification program which I'll address later.

There is no guarantee that nutritional therapy is going to work. Each body is unique and each person's situation is different. Success also depends upon how disciplined a person, (or parents) will be. The most important thing you learn right now is that there is an option. There is something constructive that you can do. You don't have to sit and allow the doctors to call the shots and order the chemotherapy and radiation treatments. I've talked to hundreds of people who have tried nutritional therapy because conventional therapies have given up on them, and they have been successful. I have met more people that have damage from surgery, radiation and chemotherapy and they are living with damage to vital organs after a course of conventional cancer treatment. Now they have vital organs that are permanently damaged and are not as responsive to nutritional therapy as they should be.

Basically, you need to ask yourself what makes sense. Chemotherapy burns the body from the inside out in hopes to destroy the cancer cells, but it also destroys the body's healthy cells and puts vital organs such as the heart, kidneys and liver at risk. On the other hand, nutritional therapy builds up the immune system and creates healthy cells to enable the body to fight the cancer. It not only enhances the overall health of the body, but also makes the body's vital organs, stronger so they can help with the detoxification process.

3

Drug Therapy vs. Nutrition: The difference between masking the symptom and curing the disease

For people who are facing a cancer diagnosis, my concern is that they understand they have options. They can decide whether to pursue nutritional therapy or the conventional therapies; chemo, radiation, and surgery. It's important to weigh both options before deciding, and to consider using a combination of both kinds of treatment. It is important to note that the reoccurence rate of cancer is over 50% for those who chose conventional therapy. I'll share some significant points of view on conventional therapy from advocates of nutritional therapy, and thoughts on our experience with Andrew's treatments, both conventionally and nutritionally.

Harold Harper, M.D. says, "The use of radiation or poison (chemotherapy) in the effort to get at the actual malignant cells is the equivalent of turning a blow torch on a wart." Also these therapies when used together, can cause serious damage to the immune system which is exactly the opposite of what nutritional therapy does.

I've watched many children in the hospital during our stays there with Andrew. I learned that surgery alone can deplete your immune system by 50%. That's why after surgery, a patient needs to stay on antibiotics for such a long time. It's because their immune system is shot. Typically, when people go into the hospital for drug therapy or surgeries, they get sick with something else before they can go home. The treatments wear down their immune system and they are vulnerable to the diseases they are exposed to in the hospital. You may recall that following Andrew's first round of chemo, he developed double-pneumonia.

Surgery is a good option to consider in some cases. If I found a massive tumor in my abdomen, I would first begin a nutritional program to boost my immune system. I would want them to attempt to remove as much of the tumor as they could, but then I would go home and continue building up my immune system nutritionally. It may be the best move to get started fighting the disease. If you have a tumor that has cancer cells multiplying at a frightening rate, you are asking a lot for your immune system to catch up after the cancer has had so long to develop. Surgery to remove a tumor may give your body a bit of a head start.

I am not a health professional, but I would suggest that maybe one or two rounds of chemo and radiation would be the best first move for people just to stun the cancer initially, to give the body time to build up its immune system through nutrition. In *A Cancer Battle Plan* Dr. Kurt W. Donsbach is quoted, "There is a place, of course, for surgery or careful and selective radiation at times and in certain forms of extremely malignant and fulminating (explosively growing) cancers, the extremely careful use of chemotherapy." He goes on to say, "None of these modalities (surgery, radiation and chemo) are effective in restoring health. They are merely suppressive and at times help to take a load off the natural immune system of the body." Cancer is basically a symptom of a weakened and degenerating body. If you are going to beat the disease, you must begin to reverse the degeneration process through detoxification and nutritional therapy. Ann Wigmore who wrote *Hippocrates Diet and Health Program* states, "Food as our medicine usually effects the body much more slowly than modern drugs, but in the end it can be safer and more thorough. It works by removing the cause of the illness whereas most drugs merely relieve the outer symptoms."

The bottom line is that drug therapy treats symptoms of cancer, not causes, while nutritional therapy treats the cause and the symptoms eventually disappear. Dr. Harper writes in *How You Can Beat the Killer Diseases*, "What if cancer is a systemic, chronic metabolic disease of which lumps and

bumps constitute only symptoms? Will this not mean that
billions of dollars have been misspent and that the basic
premise of which cancer treatment and research are grounded
are wrong? Of course it will and in decades to come, a
perplexed future generation will look back in amazement on
how current medicine approached cancer with a cobalt
machine, a surgical knife and the introduction of poisons into
the system and wonder if such brutality really occurred."
That reminds me of the story of how our first president,
George Washington was said to have died. He apparently died
at the hands of a medical doctor, because of a therapy that was
believed in back then. He had a wart, and to treat those they
would cut them out and do some bloodletting, a common
medical practice in those days. George Washington bled to
death. We look back at that and think it's not only barbaric,
but foolish. I think we will look back on today's conventional
cancer treatments and realize that chemo and radiation were
indeed barbaric practices.

My hope for the future of nutritional health care in
America is that we will bridge the gap between drug therapy
and nutritional therapy, making nutritional therapy the first
option for treating illness. I agree that drug therapy is
necessary in many cases, especially for emergency medical
care and trauma, but I would like to see a day when
nutritional therapy with quality *natural* supplements will be
covered by insurance companies. Because of the decline in
the nutritional value of foods produced in this country,
supplements are essential for fighting disease and maintaining
our health. We simply do not produce food with enough
nutrients in it to sustain optimum health. Therefore, I believe
we need to ensure that we provide our people with an
affordable way to preserve their health through the use of
nutritional supplements and organically grown foods.

In the beginning, I only knew some basic key points,
but it was enough to start with. We all have cancer cells, our
body has the ability to fight disease, and nutritional therapy
treats the cause not the symptoms. When we began Andrew's
treatment there were no terrible side effects. There are only
"side benefits" of nutritional therapy. Our quality of life
improved most considerably. We had time at home with
Andrew and the other children, because we were not at the
hospital, and that lessened the stress on the whole family. We

were ultimately able to build up Andrew's immune system and we saw test results that proved it after 90 days of nutritional treatment.

4

Detoxification:
Cleansing the body from
the inside out

When beginning to treat a degnerative disease, you
need to cleanse and detoxify the vital organs, particularly the
colon and liver. Detoxification of the body is critical when
you are trying to build an up immune system. It is probably
the most important thing a person can do in their fight against
a degenerative disease.   Our liver is very important for
detoxification. We need to support the liver because it has a
lot of jobs in the body. One of the most important is that it
aids in digestion and assimilation of nutrients and foods.
Also, it's a filtering system for harmful substances. Harold
Manner, Ph.D., professor of biology at Loyola University in
Chicago, says "Where there is cancer, it's a sure bet that it was
proceeded by a poorly functioning liver. It is one of the
body's chief organs for the elimination and conversion of
toxic substances. The livers of cancer patients become
clogged with many of the poisons that they were meant to
eliminate. Cancer can be reversed and controlled only if we
regenerate the liver. Fortunately for us, the liver is the one
organ in the body that is capable of regenerating itself. We
must immediately institute a program of purification."
Simply drinking some warm lemon water in the
morning before getting out of bed will help the liver detoxify
or, detoxifying the entire body can be done through a juice
fast combined with cleansing enemas daily, however, there are

more intense programs such as the one outlined in *A Cancer Battle Plan* written by Dave and Anne Frahm.

With Andrew, we chose not to do enemas or colonics because of his age. At first he didn't have much of an appetite, but he drank so much of the organic juice, he actually was on a juice fast and detoxifying, although we didn't realize it then. We didn't know the value of detoxifying the body yet, it just happened. For myself though, I would go full force with detoxification tomorrow if I was told that I had cancer today. A detoxifying and nutrition program is vital. Once the body is detoxified and cleansed, it will be able to use the quality nutrients it gets through quality natural food supplements and organically grown foods to heal itself. The body is designed to do it.

There are liver detoxification diets, there are coffee enemas and lemon juice enemas and water purge enemas. In *Healthy Healing* by Linda Rector-Page, Ph. D, says, "Coffee enemas have become standard in natural healing when liver and blood-related cancers are present. Caffeine used in this way stimulates the liver and gallbladder to remove toxins, open the bile ducts and encourages increased peristaltic action. It also produces the necessary enzyme activity for healthy red blood cell formation and oxygen uptake." Rector-Page also has a good example of a liver detoxification diet in her book. You can do the enemas yourself in the privacy of your own bathroom. You can get an enema kit at a drug store and it's a very simple procedure. Anne Frahm describes a two-week detoxification program which I followed for seven days and I experienced exactly what should happen as you detoxify. I felt sluggish and worn out for the first 3-4 days. By the seventh day though, I felt radiant, even pure. I looked radiant and felt alive. I had even lost some weight!

We didn't do enemas with Andrew, but I feel now that we should have. It would have helped his body with the detoxification process. He needed a big detoxification process to clean out his body after eating such a poor diet and having the chemotherapy and radiation treatments. Thankfully, through juices and vitamins, his body was able to turn over, but I think that it would have been a lot easier on his system had we regularly done some form of enema for detoxification. Dr. Paavo Airola writes in *How To Get Well*, "During fasting, a huge amount of morbid matter, dead cells and diseased tissue are burned and the toxic wastes which have been accumulated in the tissue for years causing disease and premature aging are loosened and expelled from the system. These wastes are eliminated from the system by way of kidney, bowels, skin and lungs, but the eliminatory canal, the bowel, is the main route by which the toxins are thrown out of the body. Since, during fasting, the natural bowel movements cease to take place, the toxic waste would have no way to leave the system except with the help of enemas." He goes on to say, "If you fast without enemas, these toxins remain in the system and are reabsorbed into the system, poisoning the whole body. Your body will try to get them out by other eliminative organs, particularly through the kidneys which will often be overloaded and even damaged."

The type of fasting that we have seen to be most effective is a juice fast with water and coffee enemas daily if an intense detoxification is desired. I would highly encourage people to educate themselves with the resources I've noted and pursue an aggressive detoxification program if they are dealing with a serious health problem like cancer.

5

What are we eating and why? The real effects of meat and dairy products in the body

A lot of people ask us what we have eliminated from our diet as a result of Andrew's nutritional treatment. I tell them everything white: white sugar, white flour, dairy, salt and also meat. They ask "What do you eat?" My husband's response is, "Pasta, pizza, tacos, hotdishes, stir-fries." Of course, they say it sounds like what they eat, and we answer with, "It is the same thing that you eat, only the ingredients are different. They are better for you. They are organic or natural forms of foods, rather than foods that have chemical preservatives and pesticides, additives, red dyes, etc." Learning the how's and what's of an organic whole foods diet was tough, but the adjustments have had many, many pleasing results. We'd never go back! It takes a lifestyle change, but if you can do this, you have the power to change your future and future generations of your family. You can break the chains of poor diet and eating habits by starting quality diet and eating habits today, so that your children will grow up and learn good habits vs. the high fat and high sugar diets that most Americans are accustomed to.

Most importantly for the cancer patient to eliminate from their diet is meat and dairy products. We can get all the protein and calcium we need from fresh fruits, vegetables, and raw nuts. Few of us are taught that our bodies build their own protein from the things we eat, whether it's animal protein or plant products. The body breaks it down to amino acids which produce human protein. In other words, you don't automatically get usable protein by eating it. It all depends upon how easily the food can be broken down into amino acid components. In *A Cancer Battle Plan,* Dave & Anne Frahm state, "If you eat any fruits and vegetables, nuts or sprouts on a regular basis, you are receiving all the amino acids necessary for your body to build the protein it needs." Specifically, foods that contain all eight essential amino acids, include bananas, beans, brussel sprouts, cabbage and carrots, and cauliflower, corn and cucumbers, and nuts and peas, potatoes and sesame seeds, sunflower seeds, sweet potatoes, tomatoes. All these are included in a vegetarian diet and provide the necessary amino acids that produce the protein you need. Unfortunately, even vegetarians may not get enough of these foods to provide all the protein they need. A good source is a soy-based protein supplement containing all eight essential amino acids.

If you are reluctant to switch to a vegetarian diet, consider pork products, for example. Pigs don't sweat, and the reason their meat is so salty tasting is because that's where the toxins are stored in their body. It's what the animal can't detoxifiy. Or, when you eat liver for example, you eat something from an animal's body that has spent it's time detoxifying the blood of that animal. You don't know what has gone through that piece of meat. Also, a lot our meat products come from animals that have been given antibiotics and hormones which are passed on to us when we consume them.

The human body is very adaptable, but cow's milk isn't designed for humans. Harvey and Marylin Diamond report that "over 98% of the American population is lactose intolerant." Osteoporosis patients think they need more calcium, and so include more milk, cheese and dairy in their diet. Ironically, they are actually draining their bodies of calcium. Milk and cheese turn extremely acidic in our bodies. To neutralize this acidity, our body has to alkalize the acid using calcium from our own bones. So when the calcium comes from dairy, the resulting acidity strips the calcium from the bones. The people with osteoporosis are those that have had a high dairy content in their diet. Their bodies compensate by stripping the calcium from the bones making them thinner and vulnerable to fractures.   Also, meat and dairy both expend more energy for the body to digest.   That energy is taken away from your body's ability to heal itself.

Dale and Kathy Martin in their book, *Living Well* remark that the fat in meat and dairy products "...is the most likely storage facility of pollutants from our environment.   As we eat upward on the food chain from root vegetables to grains, fruits, leafy vegetables, vegetable oils and fats, the concentration of pesticides and chemical pollutants gradually increases.   Dairy products give us a 250% increase of pollutant concentration over leafy vegetables and a 1500% increase over eating root vegetables. With the consumption of red meat, fish and poultry, the percentages already cited double.   Fat is the storage place of all the production chemicals that are being put into animals to make them grow bigger, faster.   By eating their meat,   you and I ingest concentrated amounts of hormones, antibiotics and other agents that do harm to our systems."   The fat we get from meat and dairy products is just not good for us.

A much better source of calcium is raw sesame seeds. We sprinkle them on our salads. Also all leafy greens, prunes and dates. A glass of fresh juice made from apples, carrots and spinach is a great source of calcium and betacarotene. Raw nuts are an excellent source of calcium and protein, but they are a concentrated form of those nutrients and they demand a great deal for your body to digest because of their form.   With Andrew our objective was to rebuild his body in the first stages of his healing, so we did not allow the raw nuts until his body was at a point where he could handle it.

When he was diagnosed, Andrew's diet was very poor. He ate a lot of dairy which is very mucous-forming and cancer feeds on mucous.   I wasn't aware that I was actually feeding the cancer in his body. Andrew was in the process of dying and very uncomfortable.   The first thing we eliminated was the milk in his bottle and we introduced the organic carrot-apple juice. We weaned him by juicing more apples than carrots and then slowly added more carrots. By the grace of God, Andrew loved it and that step was easy. We pursued that wholeheartedly trying to get as much into him as possible, up to six eight-ounce bottles a day.

Nutritionist Anne Wigmore wrote, "Nature's plan called for food enzymes to help with digestion instead of

forcing the body's own digestive enzymes to carry the whole
load." After a good detoxification process the liver needs a
break. We needed to take the load off Andrew's liver by
feeding him foods that had a lot of enzymes. Living foods
are foods with live enzymes. Plant and animal foods both
have enzymes in their natural state, but when food is cooked,
these enzymes are lost. Heat destruction of enzymes begins at
107 degrees farenheit. In the Frahm's book, Dave illustrates,
"Suppose that tomorrow morning you were to go out to your
car only to find someone had walked off with your spark
plugs. Without them your car is dead, right? Enzymes do for
your body what spark plugs do for your car. Without them,
nothing else can happen." Marie Salaman, a nutritionist
agrees, she calls them "catalysts." Dr. Mary Swope referred
to them as "a 'life force' in maintaining health and healing."
Dave Frahm writes, "Enzymes supply the energy for all the
biochemical reactions upon which life is built, including the
digestion of food. Our bodies have digestive enzymes, and
they are reactivated by the liver. The impact of a poorly
functioning liver upon the entire body is obvious. Reduced
enzyme activity leads to poor digestion, which leads to
undernourished cells, and in this state, the body's immune
system falters. Organs begin to become dysfunctional and
disease is imminent."

        At a health seminar I attended in 1995 a doctor from
the Mayo Clinic said, "People, we are eating dead food, and
that's why we are dying of degenerative diseases." In our
country, more than 90% of the enzymes in milk are destroyed
by pasteurization. About 65% of foods in our grocery stores
are processed or refined, so their enzymes are destroyed. By
the time whole grain rice is turned into a quick-cooking
"instant" rice, it loses 75% of it's nutrients. We really are
eating dead, worthless food in this country. I remember
someone telling me we need to remember that in the
beginning, we were placed in a Garden, not a fast-food
restaurant!

        In addition to the dead food we eat, our fresh fruits
and vegetables have been sprayed with chemicals and
pesticides. It's almost impossible to remove them by washing
because as they grow, it becomes an internal problem. You
can't wash that off. In my own research and education I
learned that by the time they put a carrot on the shelf at the

supermarket, it has been sprayed, on the average at least 14 times with pesticides.

Max Gerson, M.D. wrote in *A Cancer Therapy*, "The coming years will make it more and more important that organically grown fruit and vegetables will be and must be used for protection against degenerative diseases, the prevention of cancer and moreso, the treatment of cancer." It's the way that we are eating that causes us to see a rise in cancer and other degenerative diseases. Americans are under stress, therefore their bodies are under stress. If we don't give our immune system the proper nutrition it needs to fight with our environment, we will continue to see more illness in the future. This is why it's important to consume only whole, organic foods. Organic foods are foods made with produce that hasn't been sprayed with pesticides or treated with chemical fertilizers. Whole foods are those that have not been cooked to the point where all the enzymes are killed and nutrients are lost. When food is overcooked, it's ruined, and weakened and our bodies cannot use it.

When cooking food, it's best to use glass, stainless steel or even surgical stainless steel cookware. Aluminum and teflon-coated cookwares should not be used, because these elements can come off into the food and your body can absorb dangerous amounts of it over time.

A cookbook I recommend for getting started is *Lifestyle for Health, Smart Cooking for Busy People*, by Cheryl Townsely. I have looked at a lot of cookbooks and this is a good one. It has strategies, recipes, and a calender. For instance, she gives a list for what to buy for the month of May, and then what to cook for the month of May. The recipes are easy and quick and your family will like them. She has published other cookbooks too, including one for children. She gives brand names to use in the recipes and they really work.

Making the switch to veganism, (no meat, dairy, or sugar) after education was not a hard choice for us. At first, you might think you have to give up a lot and it doesn't sound very attractive, but the more you educate yourself about what you eat now, the more you become willing to do it. Danny Vierra has a ministry called Modern Manna. He educates people about how to follow a vegan diet and what some of the truths are about meat protein and dairy. His resources are easily understood and excellently produced. I would encourage anyone considering a vegetarian or vegan diet to get his information.

Getting the children to cooperate with our plan was difficult at first. We simply put the new foods in front of them and let them know that was it. There were no other choices. When they didn't want to try something new,   we used phrases like, "This is the plan." and "You need to obey."

When it comes to foods that their friends are allowed to eat, like fried foods, candy, or anything processed, we tell them, "It's not a part of our diet." The older kids understood that we were changing our diet in support of Andrew, and the little ones just followed along. We explained to them very specifically, the reasons for eliminating meat, dairy and sugar from our diet. Of course, they didn't always like the idea of eating mostly raw, fresh fruits and vegetables, but over time, they became accustomed to the fact that it was all there was to eat and they complied. It was a process and it took a lot of patience and diligence on the part of David and I. You can do it too, just don't expect it to happen overnight!

A vegetarian diet allows your body to produce all the protein you need, but at the same time you are avoiding the fat and the excessive protein found in animal fats. Fat is essential for good nutrition, but too much fat can be cancer-causing. If you cut out animal fat from meat and dairy products the fat in your diet will come down to acceptable levels. There is a difference between good fats and bad fats. Bad fats are carcinogenic, or cancer-causing. Fats that have been heat processed, such as in fried foods, are highly carcinogenic. Hydrogenated fats have been heat processed. Oils should be unrefined and cold pressed. Extra virgin olive oil is an example of a good kind of fat along with avocados. Anne Frahm suggests an alternative for butter which is made by mixing one cup canola oil with two sticks of real butter in the blender. Keep it refrigerated and use it sparingly.

Another significant factor in the diet of the cancer patient is fiber. Fiber is found in whole grains and fruits and vegetables. They need to consume whole grain breads, not just wheat bread. Fiber is important for the body's colon function and detoxification, and it is essential for fighting cancer. It helps clear the colon, allowing the body to remove toxins. It aids the growth of friendly intestinal bacteria and helps with absorption and assimilation of the nutrients that we give ourselves through nutritional therapy. We got a daily fiber mix for Andrew and we put it in everything in his diet that we could. We used a type that could be mixed with juice, sprinkled on toast, or even added to a bread or hotdish recipe.

We also included a green drink in Andrew's diet. We found Kyo-Green to be the best product offered. The ingredients are wheat grass, young barley leaves, kelp and blue-green algea, chlorophyll, and brown rice. It's a great blood builder, oxygenator and free radical scavenger. We added it to Andrew's juices as an important part of his daily protocol. You can also add some fresh spinach juice to carrot-apple juice making a great fresh green drink full of calcium, vitamins and live-enzymes.

We have talked to many people all across the country who have heard about our story and have inquired about what we did for Andrew. All who have made the changes we've suggested have seen dramatic results in the quality of their lives. Not only do they feel better emotionally and physically, but mentally too. You too, can begin to feel more alert, and more alive. With determination, cancer patients and their families can confidently embrace a hope they may not have had with conventional therapy.

6

Essential Supplements
for fighting cancer,
including Andrew's protocol

Unfortunately, we cannot get all the nutrients we need from our food and we are bombarded daily with toxins in our air and water. Poor air, soil and water quality lead to poor food quality and no matter how nutrition conscious we become, we still will be unable to get all the things that we need from eating right alone. Including pure, natural supplements in the diet can help build up the body's immune system. Natural food supplements are pure, organic foods that are cold-processed and concentrated into a tablet or capsule form.

The fiber mix and the Kyo-green products are only some of the food supplements we used in Andrew's protocol. Let me share what I know about the other supplements we used:

Betacarotene, also known as vitamin A, was the most important supplement we started with. It is an excellent antioxidant and is able to combat free radicals that cause cancer in the body. Betacarotene is turned into vitamin A by the liver as the body needs it. It helps to ensure cell growth and makes sure cells mature and live to do what they're supposed to do. You can get plenty of betacarotene in carrot juice, which was a big part of Andrew's protocol. Betacarotene is an effective agent in stimulating the immune system to protect the body. It's fat soluble and unlike synthetic vitamin A, it does not reach toxic levels in the body because the liver converts it to vitamin A only as it's needed. In *How To Fight Cancer and Win*, William Fisher notes the beneficial qualities of betacarotene. He says, "As both a preventative and an active cancer treatment, betacarotene has been shown to effectively destroy the cancer cells protective layering of mucous, opening it to the body's natural defense mechanism. Proponents of betacarotene predict a reduction in the rate of certain forms of cancer for those who regularly include carrots in their diet. (Up to 80% of cancer in the lungs and bronchia and up to 55% of the cancer in the colon.)"

B-complex is helpful for healing hearts and to stimulate the immune system. It inhibits the growth of tumors and cancer cells. It is water soluble and is the first to be used up when your body's under stress. Your body is continually under stress when you have cancer. Even if you are calm on the outside, your body is still carrying the burden of fighting cancer on the inside. Andrew seemed to be calm and didn't show a lot of stress emotionally, but his body was definately feeling the effects of the battle, so B-complex was a significant part of his protocol. Incidentally, it's noted as the "happy" vitamin, it regulates your blood sugar, and is great for PMS, depression, and migraine headaches.

Vitamin C. The absence of vitamin C puts you at a risk for cancer. Therefore, vitamin C is a very important supplement in fighting this disease. Dave and Anne Frahm call it "the big gun." It inhibits cancer and is one of the most potent antioxidants known. Patrick Quillin concluded "that vitamin C stimulates the immune system to attack the newly sprouted abnormal cells, it is a free radical scavenger, mopping up free radicals to prevent destruction of the DNA. It stimulates the production of interferon, a potent anti-cancer agent in the body. It blocks the formation of carcinogenic nitrosamines in the stomach." Linus Pauling, Ph.D., who has spent years researching vitamin C and it's effects says, "With the properties of vitamin C for cancer, we could cut the death rate by 70 %. This would be 70% of 650,000 people who die every year of cancer." Obviously, a high intake of vitamin C is beneficial to all cancer patients.

Vitamin E, like vitamin A, is fat soluble. When used with the trace mineral selenium the anti-cancer properties of both are enhanced. Like vitamin C, E is thought to hinder the production of cancer-causing compounds in the stomach and the intestines. It's an antioxidant that hunts down the free-radicals and destroys them. It should be noted that Vitamin E should be gradually increased and people should not be started on high doses initially. Selenium also has other important properties that aid in cancer treatment: As stated in *A Cancer Battle Plan*, "At high levels it is directly toxic to cancer cells. It retards the tumors in breast tissue and can deactivate radiation toxicity in the body. It works to clean the body from the effects of chemotherapy and liver malfunction. It is a potent stimulant to the immune system. It is a powerful trace mineral. Selenium should be taken under the supervision of a health professional. It's very important to make sure other trace minerals are included in your diet as well." Andrew would get calcium magnesium, and zinc through daily food supplements.

Garlic is a powerful food. We used garlic supplements as a major part of Andrew's protocol. At times he even smelled like garlic. It stimulates the immune system's functions and also plays a role in the prevention of heart disease. It reduces serum cholesterol, blood pressure.

Alfalfa is an anti-inflammatory, and supports detoxification. Alfalfa has many qualities that are good for everyone, and this supplement was also included in Andrew's program. It helps cleanse the body and is a good remedy for hayfever allergies when taken with vitamin C everyday. We used it along with a very natural herbal laxative to help Andrew's body continually cleanse itself.

EPA, or eicosapentaenoic acid is beneficial to cancer patients because it actually protects against cancer. This is more commonly known as fish oil. It is a kind of fat, but remember, some fats in the diet are good for us. We did not use this in Andrew's protocol, only because I didn't know about it during the first years of his treatment. I see the benefits of using it now in his daily regimen.

Pure shark cartilage cuts off the blood supply to tumors. We learned about it when someone gave us a book entitled, *Sharks Don't Get Cancer*, by Dr. William Lane It's only side effect for children is that it also cuts the blood supply to healthy growing tissue, and as a result it stunts their growth. However, this is not an issue for adults who choose to use shark cartilage. Andrew is small for his age, but he is very much alive. This is the only supplement we used that had a negative side effect, and we believe the benefits far outweigh the risk here and would recommend it's use for children. As always, consult a health professional.

For reasons already discussed, we cannot possibly eat the amount of nutrients that our bodies require. Pure, natural supplements are essential. Do not buy synthetics, they are worthless. They don't break down fast enough for your body to assimilate them. You have to make sure that the company providing the supplement has done scientific research on their products. They need to be cold-water processed. If they are heated they will lose value. Also, a B-complex supplement should contain 100% biotin and 100% folic acid vs. a ratio like 4% biotin and 2000 % Thymus in a lot of cheaper B-complexes on the market. B's work like a family and they need to be in sync with one another. Biotin and folic acid are the most expensive B-vitamins to manufacture, so even though a company might say their supplements are all natural, they might leave out necessary amounts of these nutrients. Also, they only need to be 10% natural to say that they are a "natural" product. I challenge you to do your research. Refuse to be a victim of the frauds and ask for advice from people that are knowledgable about this kind of a program.

Dr. Bruce Miller educates people on how to choose natural supplements. He shares a list of things to check for in his lecture "Five basic rules for natural supplements."
1. Make sure it has all nineteen nutrients on the RDA.
2. There should be no large percent differences in the B-vitamins as described above.
3. Biotin and Folic acid should not be left out.
4. Zinc and Copper should be in 100% ratio with RDA, from 15mg to 2mg, not smaller amounts.
5. Calcium, magnesium and phosphorous should be included. They are hard to put into a tablet form and some companies may skip them to save money.

The objective of giving megadoses of vitamins and mineral supplements in the treatment of cancer is to rebuild the healthy cells, help the body change its chemistry and to reinforce the body's own protective systems. Vitamins and minerals aid your body in it's fight to cure itself of cancer. They help restore and reinforce the body's ability to fight off disease. Dr. Joel Robbins observed, "It's the body's action and utilization of nutrients for healing, not the nutrients action on the body" that makes the difference in healing. If the body is so degenerated and weak that it cannot use the supplements you give it, you will get few results. And, you have to remember that using vitamin and mineral supplementation does not work overnight. In *Healthy Healing*, Linda Rector-Page points out that "vitamins and minerals are at the deepest levels of the body's processes and regenerative changes in the body's chemistry usually require as much time to rebuild as they did to decline." The medical community has us accustomed to getting fast results through drug therapy to relieve the symptoms of deeper illnesses. With cancer, the task is to reverse the body's downward spiral of degeneration and it takes time and energy to do that.

Generally it does take weeks to see proven results when using nutritional therapy. However, I've read case studies where it has not taken a very long time. In Anne Frahm's case, she was loaded with cancer and after five weeks of nutritional therapy, she was cancer free. Also during the writing of this book, I talked to a woman with ovarian cancer who had been left hopeless after three years of conventional treatments. After learning about Andrew's protocol she tried it for one week. She then returned to her doctor for tests and was told that for the first time in three years, her cancer cells had decreased by 1%. That's not very much of an improvement, but as she put it, "It's 1% in the right direction." People should not be fooled, there is no special hype with nutritional therapy. It is simply a matter of an extended period of time for your body to revitalize the entire chemistry and metabolism. The whole system has been heading downhill for a long time and it needs to start going up hill.

Supplements need to be balanced, and should be taken with the supervison of a natural health professional. There are so many that work together to detoxify the body and boost the immune system that the information can be overwhelming for those also under the stress of having a terminal disease. They may not have the time, or the energy to pursue this information. I encourage friends and family to come along side them and be their partner in fighting disease. Learn all you can for their sake and share the information with them at times when you sense they can handle it.

Following is Andrew's protocol in detail:

We chose Shaklee natural supplements because we believe that they are the best natural supplements offered on the market, and the only ones I know that are backed with rigorous clinical studies, research and development. Our exact protocol initially was:

- 30-50 ounces of fresh organic carrot-apple juice every day. Some we put into his G-tube, and some he drank as described earlier.
- Betacarotene 10,000 I.U. Thirty a day for the first twelve days. He took ten a day after that.
- Shaklee's adult multi-vitamin Vita-Lea, three daily.
- 500mg sustained-release Vitamin C, nine daily.
- Balanced B-complex, six daily.
- Vitamin E 400 I.U. with 10mcgs selenium, six daily.
- Zinc 15mg, three daily.
- Calcium magnesium complex, six daily.
- 500mg garlic in a tablet equivalent to one clove of garlic, six daily
- Three tablespoons of Protein three times a day.
- Pure Alfalfa tablets, fifteen daily.
- Shaklee's Herb-lax, two before bed every night.
- 100% pure shark cartilage according to his weight, three daily.
- Kyo-Dophilus, one daily. Kyo-Dophilus is a trio of friendly bacteria.
- Two teaspoons of Kyo-Green, mixed with juice or water, twice daily. Kyo-Green is a powdered green drink of barley, wheatgrass and fine kelp.
- Fiber mix, 1 tsp in the vitamin-juice mixture that went into his tube, three times a day.

Max Gerson says, "In general people go to hospitals for operations or serious illnesses, and the family considers them recovered upon return. This is different with cancer. Cancer is a degenerative disease, not an acute one and the treatment can be an effective one only if carried out strictly in accordance with the rules for one and a half to two years. It is not a symptom that is treated, nor a specific disease, but the reactions and functions of the entire body which have to be transformed and restored." Remember, it takes discipline to be consistent with this kind of treatment. You are in charge. I know that one or two years may seem like a long time, but it's worth a lifetime. You can do it!

7

Mission Impossible:
Maintaining a positive attitude

Exercise. If a person is dealing with cancer, they need to start an exercise program slowly. With Andrew we didn't start a special exercise program because he was active and had a lot of energy when he was feeling well. Generally, it's not a big issue for children. For an adult, however, not only does it help you maintain emotional well-being, but your body needs to have a little physical exertion, and regular exercise supports your body's overall ability to function. In *Getting Well Again*, Dr. Carl Simonton and his wife, Stephanie, who help cancer patients recover from the disease note that their patients who were physically active had the best recoveries. There are certain limitations, however. Dr. Simonton suggests that even patients with special conditions like cancer in the bone and low platelet counts can proceed very slowly with an exercise program. They just need to be very careful and pay close attention to warning signs like pain and stiffness.

Keeping a positive attitude. When we were first told what we had to undertake nutritionally for Andrew, I felt good about something that we could do to help him. The information was overwhelming. but it all made so much sense. I felt better emotionally because I was doing something *constructive* and fighting for him. God designed a miraculous body with the ability to do amazing things. It was very rewarding to take part in supporting that body towards wellness.

We took the time to make sure there were a lot of positive affirmations, laughter and fun in Andrew's life. We invited people over that he loved to be around. They would do fun things with him and tickle him and he would giggle. We still sit down on the floor and tickle Andrew, calling it his medicine. We call it laugh therapy. We considered it a very important part of his treatment because it's so beneficial to the body. It releases tension and stress. Norman Cousins wrote, "Some people in the grip of uncontrollable laughter say their ribs are hurting. The expresssion is probably accurate, but it is a delightful hurt that leaves the individual relaxed almost to the point of an open sprawl. It is the kind of pain too, that most people would do well to experience everyday of their lives. It is as specific and tangible as any other form of exercise. Though its biochemical manifestations have as yet to be as implicitly charted as the effects of fear or frustration or rage, they are real enough."

When well-meaning doctors make mistakes because of their ignorance of nutritional therapy or their bias toward conventional therapies for cancer we must forgive them. It has helped my husband and I to base our forgiveness and love toward them on biblical principles. It has also been important to strengthen our spiritual and emotional being through Scripture. So many people told us to have faith in God and quoted bible verses to us like Romans 3:23, "God works all things together for the good of those who love him, for those who are called according to his purpose." Which is a great verse, but not very comforting when your are watching your child waste away before your eyes. We were told to trust God and that He wouldn't give us what we couldn't handle. I would get so angry. I wanted to respond by saying, "Oh Yeah? Well, I've had enough. I've told God that I've had *enough.*" The turning point for me was when I realized what God was willing to do to bring unity between he and I. He was willing to let his only Son be tortured and hung on a cross so that someday I could be with him, safe in heaven. I finally felt his arms of love and saw a glimpse of his character that day rocking Andrew in his hospital room. God is very unselfish. When I became intimately acquainted with him, faith was much easier to come by and my trust in him to take care of Andrew and our family became much stronger. It was more real, but I had to have that time alone with him and get to know him. That lesson in the hospital had a profound affect on me. It helped maintain my morale and helped me to deal with things better. There were times when I was angry and tired of watching Andrew's suffering, but there came a point when I had to surrender to God. I don't mean that I had to get on my knees and beg him. He's not a taskmaster. In *Coronary? Cancer? God's Answer: Prevent It!*, Dr. Richard Brennan puts it this way, "To ignore God at any time in one's life is a foolishness I find difficult to understand. To ignore him while staring sickness and disease in the face is more than foolish." I feel that God is calling us during those difficult times. He doesn't cause them, but he longs for us to ask for his help, admitting that we cannot fight this terrible "giant" alone. One of the most effective things you can do as a cancer patient or as someone supporting the patient is to ask for God's help.

Apart from personal encouragement from God and His Word, the most important thing that David and I did for our mental attitude in dealing with this disease was to play "The Glad Game". It's from the movie *Pollyanna*. Whatever situation we found ourselves in, whether we were having to be in the hospital longer than we expected, or were stretched financially once again, we would try to play "The Glad Game." We thought of anything we could be glad about within the situation. There was always something, but we had to have the right heart and state of mind to find it.

You're in charge. Another way a cancer patient or their family members can improve their morale within the situation is to realize that with nutritional therapy you have better control. You can take initiative and begin to do constructive things to fight the disease. When our son Jake was fourteen months old he was critically ill in the hospital. We stayed with him all the time and had not gone home for months. Finally, we decided it would be best for us to go home one night and leave Jake. We did and were called at 4 a.m. They told us that Jake was in trouble and they didn't think he was going to make it through the night. We had to get to the hospital. They said that Jake was tachycardic and that his heart was beating about 150 beats per minute. I had to go alone because David decided he should check in at work first. He was so afraid of losing his job and we were already uncomfortably financially strapped.

When I walked into the room, I saw Jake's chest heaving in and out. He only weighed about 14 pounds and was very pale. There was a resident, an intern and a nurse standing there. They all looked very grave. It appeared to be a tense situation, not only because of Jake's condition, but they were all visibly frustrated with one another. It became apparent quickly that the resident and intern had been arguing. The intern had a syringe in his hand and he was shaking his head when I walked in as if to say "No." The resident was standing there glaring at him and said, "Give it to me, and I will give it to him." I said, "What's going on?" The nurse said, "There's a drug that they want to give Jake that they think will help him to calm his heart down, but the intern doesn't feel comfortable with it because we have been giving him a lot of things, and he's afraid that the mixture will push him over the edge." The resident said, "Enough of that, just give it to me and I will do it." The intern kept hold of the syringe and said, "No, I'm not going to do it." It was almost as if they were going to get into a fist fight. I sat down on the heat register and looked at Jake. I didn't know what to think and I was scared. They continued to bicker back and forth. Finally, the nurse looked me straight in the eye and she said, "Leanne, you have control over this situation." It was the first time that somebody said that I had an option. I was in charge. I looked at the resident and I said, "No more drugs. Get out of the room." He stormed off, barking at the nurse and intern to follow him. They proceeded to go out into the hallway and continued arguing with each other.

Later, I found out that the resident was fired. After all, I was left alone in the room with a child who was critically ill. I was crying and sobbing because it had all been too much for me to bear. I was praised by a lot of people on the floor that day because of the proactive stance I'd taken in Jake's health care. It was a valuable lesson for me to learn when it came time to deal with Andrew's cancer. I knew that it was David and I who called the shots. The doctors were hired by us.

I wasn't intimidated anymore after that. That night they took Jake out of the main floor and put him into intensive care. They simply eliminated the drugs, turned down the lights and kept the movement to a minimum. A nurse and I sat quietly by his bedside and barely talked. Occasionally, we looked at each other and would glance up at the monitors and we watched him slowly improve and decline and if his blood pressure got low, she would move and fidget as if to run and call for help. We kept it as quiet as possible and within five days, Jake stabilized and left intensive care.

8

Creating a network of
health professionals

It's important for people to consult with a nutritionist or some kind of medical advisor, but there is a fine line, because it is also important for them to take the bulk of responsibility for their health into their own hands. There are no guarantees either way. You cannot depend solely on a professional to heal you. You must do the work. Nutritional therapy provides your body with the opportunity to build the immune system. If you have questions or doubts about it, read and educate yourself. Rather than just trusting someone else, continue to ask if it makes sense. Try it. Natural supplements are not going to hurt you. But you will have to do some homework and question the products to find out which ones are the best. Charles Simone, M.D. is an oncologist trying to bridge the gap between drug therapy and nutritional therapy. In *Cancer and Nutrition*, he writes, "Good health does not come easily, you must work for it."

You need to get the facts about what you are going to put into your body. You need to find a nutritionist, which is someone trained specifically in nutritional therapy. A dietician is not trained about detoxification or the use of supplements in nutritional therapy. Typically, cancer patients will be educated in a hospital by a dietician. I would go to the hospital and walk on the floors and watch the kids that were dying from cancer. They would be given a lot of fat, sugar and low fiber foods. Doctors want them to get the pounds on during chemotherapy, because it usually causes weight loss. Increasing their weight is not health. That shows an outdated mentality on the part of dieticians and medical doctors. Cancer patients should be eating fresh salads and drinking carrot-apple juice to stimulate the immune system and their liver functions. Dieticians offer chocolate chip cookies, soft drinks, french fries and pizzas. Most people are not willing to change their diets to a healthier one, but if they knew that a healthy change in their diet might help them to conquer cancer, they may become willing to cut out the foods that are killing them. Richard Brennan, M.D. says, "What a world of good nurses could accomplish if they were better informed about the nutritional way to combat disease." Medical doctors and nurses today are not trained in nutritional therapy. Andrew's oncologist admitted to me that she was given about 55 minutes of nutritional education in her curriculum.

Nutritionists are the experts in the field of nutritional therapy. They are trained in the detoxification of the body and can educate you regarding fasting and bowel cleansing. They are also knowledgable about which foods or food supplements are needed to restore the body to optimum health. Some of them sell dietary supplements such as vitamins and minerals. Make sure you find someone who is more concerned about counseling you rather than just selling you products.

Oncologists are medical doctors who are trained in chemotherapy. It's necessary to have an oncologist on your side if you decide to undergo chemo, radiation or surgery. They can also monitor the cancer activity in your system. We continued to have lab work done on Andrew through visits with our oncologist. I valued the input that she gave even after we began nutritional therapy, and we've maintained a very healthy, positive relationship with her. Anne Frahm's oncologist said, "I can't cure you with chemotherapy, but perhaps I can keep you alive long enough for you to learn how to cure yourself." That is such an honest, humble statement. I wish all medical doctors had that attitude.

Chiropractors are trained to take care of the body's nervous system, since it controls all the other systems in the body. We sought the help of our friend and chiropractor, Dr. Pete Wurdemann. Basically, the nervous system is the fuse box to your organs and controls the functioning of your body. If a part of your nervous system is not healthy, it affects the part of the body it controls and illness can result. Chiropractors use manipulation and adjustments, especially in the spine, to make sure that the pathways for nerves and their impulses are clear and not pinched off anywhere. Dr. Wurdemann says, "My experience with Andrew has changed how I practice healthcare. Our society is obsessed with 'disease-care.' I believe that the body has the innate potential to heal naturally without drugs or surgery, but I am still amazed when I think back three years ago of Andrew and the severity of the loss of his health and how quickly he recovered with the mega-doses of supplements, chiropractic care and prayer."

Colonic Therapist. Enlisting the help of a colonic therapist is important during the detoxification process. Anne Frahm suggests picking up John M.Fink's *Third Opinion* which lists names and locators of cancer support groups. You might also try to obtain some information at your local health food store.

If you are looking for a network of physicians, Dave and Anne Frahm's "HealthQuarter's" organization provides information, education and encouragement to fellow cancer patients and educates people on nutritional therapy. They have a list of resources, doctors and health professionals where you can find support for your specific nutritional therapy.

I'd like to share with you some of my favorite quotes about selecting health professionals. Joel Robbins is a doctor of chiropractic who wrote, *Health Through Nutrition* . In his book he advises, "Do not believe in an authority, rather examine all that an authority says. Put everything to the test. Let truth be your authority, not authority your truth." Harvey and Marylin Diamond in *Fit For Life II: The Living Health Book*, say that, "No practitioner should be treated as the only and ultimate authority on health care. Each can offer the benefit of what he or she has learned but it is up to you using your common sense, instincts, past experience, and present needs and future goals to decide whether what a practitioner decides is true and helpful to you. This is how you remain in charge." Hippocrates said, "Nature made the cure, the doctor's job is to aid nature." And finally, in *Killing Cancer, The Jason Winters Story*, author Benjamin Roth Smythe writes, "Find a doctor who believes that God is greater than the medical association and you have found a jewel."

I want to leave you with two questions you should ask your doctor.

1. When prescribing medication for you, ask them, "Are you treating the symptoms or the cause of my problem?"
    Obviously, you want them to treat the cause.

2. "What do you know about the long-term side effects of this medication?
    Be cautious if they cannot give you any information, or if they shrug it off.
    I trust our experience will enlighten you and motivate you to seek natural health professionals in your program.

9

Life support:
How you can help a family fighting cancer

One of the purposes of this book is to encourage those who are fighting cancer or other degenerative diseases to take action to insure their own health. For those who are supporting people undergoing nutritional therapy I am including a simple list of practical things you can do to help them through the process. Dr. Max Gearson, in *A Cancer Therapy*, wrote "The mental condition of the patient and the psychological cooperation of the family and the environment play important roles in the restoration of the body. Every patient needs faith, love, hope and encouragement."

Even with all the support we received, there were many times that I fell apart emotionally, and in a lot of ways I fell apart spiritually, too. I want to stress the point that there is much that one can do to support a family dealing with a terminal illness. It takes the extra stress away if you will do whatever you can.

Don't ever, ever ask a family, "What can I do for you?" You cannot believe how emotionally draining that question is. It makes them have to think even more. It makes them have to mentally examine their list of overwhelming responsibilities and then make a decision. In a situation like this, they are making life-threatening decisions every day and having a difficult time doing that. So for them to have to think about what you can do for them, adds stress. It doesn't relieve it. Never ask that question.

Talk to them. Listen to them. Be in tune to what they are saying. They might say something like, "I'm so stressed, and this is getting so hard, everything is piling up. It's even overwhelming to look at the mail. And to figure out what bills to pay first, because we are just so crunched financially and the washing machine is on the fritz." They just named some things you could do for them. You could help them out financially, you could come over and organize their bills and prioritize them as far as dates and when they should pay, figuring out the minimum that they can get away with paying. You can call someone about the washing machine, or get donations for it to be fixed or replaced. You could come over, pick up their laundry and do it for them at your house. Don't ask them. Just tell them that you'll do it. You could say, "I'll come over today at 3:00 p.m. to pick up your laundry (be specific about time) and I'll return it at 7:00 p.m. folded. All you'll have to do is put it away." That's what people who are going through terminal diseases need. They don't need any questions. They just need you to tell them what you are going to do.

There's a point where it can be too much, though. If they say, "No, that's OK." Press the issue a little bit. Tell them, "No I really want to do this, it will refresh me." Then if they say, "I really don't want you to do this." and they are really adamant about it, say, "Is it really going to bug you to let me do this because it would mean a lot to me?" If they say "Yes", then don't. You can't help someone that doesn't want to be helped, but sometimes people don't even realize they need help. It could be that they don't want to accept any help because it would injure their pride. If so, just wait and try again another time.

One of the patterns I fell into during Andrew's treatments was trying to arrange everything myself. I am the eternal organizer and when I shifted into survival mode, I was determined to make everything run as smoothly as possible. I was constantly arranging babysitters so I could get Andrew to doctor visits and treatments. Unfortunately, other people have busy lives and schedules too, and could not always be there to watch my children. When I couldn't find an available sitter, I would get frustrated and angry. I did realize after some time though, that I had not been asking God to meet those needs. I had been trying to do it all through my own devices and strength, and it didn't always work. Spending time in humble, believing prayer is more effective than ten phone calls to people when you're looking for a sitter, or if there is a financial need. Know that God has made you, and he hasn't left you to handle this life with your own devices. Before you ask anyone else for help, ask Him.

Here's a list of things you can do to help:

- Stay involved in the family's life.
- Help develop a network of friends to support that person.
- Continue to be there at the low times, even though it might be awkward for you.
- Ask the cancer patient specifically how they are doing.
- Be willing to listen.
- You don't need to have the right answers. Just let them talk.
- Pray with them.
- Encourage them to pray alone.
- Encourage a group to pray for them and let them know you are doing it.
- Help the person practically with everyday chores.
- Don't tell them about your good intentions if you cannot follow through.
- Find books that will educate them about nutritional therapy and buy it for them.
- Donate money. Insurance doesn't cover good supplements and organic foods.
- Send them what you would like to receive if you were the one in need.
- Send encouraging scripture verses on convenient cards. One woman did that for me.
- Write a note telling them you care.
- Relieve the primary caretaker if you can.
- Find out what would help most by listening. Don't ask them what you can do. It's too stressful for them to always be delegating responsibilities.
- Take their other children places. They are missing out because of the illness too.

10

Spiritual Supplementation: Pure nutrition for your soul

During my first years as a young mother I had been basking in self-pity. I had a past that included sexual abuse and neglect. I was a single mom at age 19. I was forced to give up my career because of Jake's illness. I had to learn how to take care of oxygen, feeding tubes, Hickman's and Heparin locks. They said Jake wouldn't live past a year and we lost so much of our lives in the hospital. I resented being forced to deal with these things, and felt I was losing more and more control over my life. I became very bitter about all of it. Then Andrew was diagnosed. I know that we all have some kind of pain from our past that we try to soothe, but I thought this was too much, it wasn't fair. I wanted some encouragement from God, some reason for all this to be happening.

I came to the realization that God is not a taskmaster, nor is he a puppet. In Hannah Whitall Smith's book, *The Unselfishness of God,* she writes, "I saw that He was not only my saviour for the future, but that God was my significant saviour for the present. He was my captain to fight my battles for me. In order that I need not fight the battles myself, he was my burden-bearer to carry my burdens in order that I might roll them off my own weak shoulders, and give them to him. He was my fortress to hide me from my enemies and my shield to protect me, and my guide to lead me, my comforter to console me, my shepherd to care for me and no longer did I need to care for, protect or fight for myself, it was all in the hands of the one who was mighty to save and what I could do was but to trust him."

It's so important to know the One you are trusting in. You cannot get to know someone simply by hearing about them and believing they exist. You have to spend time with them. You have to talk to them. You get to a point when you are comfortable enough to be vulnerable and then you can share more of yourself. A relationship with God is like that. Getting to know him requires that you talk to him, tell him your needs, ask him to show you who he is. He won't disappoint you in that.

Christian artist, Rich Mullins sings a song that I like. Some of the lyrics in it are, "You meet the Lord in the furnace, a long time before you meet him in the sky." I can identify with that because I feel like I've been in a furnace for a long time. It's where I did finally meet God and come to rely on him for everything. I'm anxious now to meet him in the sky!

Hannah Whitall Smith says, "The Almighty God, the Creator of Heaven and Earth is not a far off God, dwelling in a heaven of unapproachable glory, but has come down in Christ to dwell with us right here in this world, in the midst of our poor ignorant helpless lives as close to us as we are to ourselves. If we believe in Christ at all, we are shut up to believing this, for this is his name, God with us." Immanuel is one of the names for Jesus Christ. It means literally, 'God with us'. I had to come to understand that God was truly with me, but first I had to get rid of the pain from the past and even my present circumstances.

When I accepted Christ for my salvation in 1989, it was a major turning point. It still didn't answer the questions of why my family and I had to go through so much until I'd heard about a family in our church whose young son had cancer. Andrew had not yet been diagnosed, but Jake was still on oxygen and feeding tubes at the time. We were out of the hospital more at that point than in with him and we felt more stabilized. I had the opportunity to sit down one night and pray about what to share with her. I wrote a note to her that was about three pages long and it took me until three in the morning. I cried and sobbed after I finished because I realized that the only reason that I could write anything that would support and encourage her was because I knew what it was like to have a terminally ill child. I was in the midst of it with Jake. It felt so good to have something tangible to share with someone else that would be helpful. It felt so refreshing in my spirit and my soul to turn around and build someone up and encourage them during a hard time. The only reason I could do it effectively was because I had walked down that road. The circumstances are different, but the pain and the fear are the same. 2Corinthians 1:3-4 says, "Praise be to the God and Father of our Lord Jesus Christ, the Father of compassion and the God of all comfort, who comforts us in all our troubles, so that we can comfort those in any trouble with the comfort we ourselves have received from God."   This verse was so true for me at that moment, when I was able to relax a little about Jake's health and encourage someone else. Although, I am sure I would not have been comforted much if someone had quoted that to me in the midst of the scary times by saying something like, "It's all in God's plan, Leanne. God is doing this so that one day you'll be able to comfort others."   It's not very encouraging to hear that you're suffering so that one far off day you will be able to help someone else. Weeks after I sent that letter to them, they both approached me at church and said, "You don't know how encouraging your letter has been to us. It has helped us so much." The boy's father told me that he read it several times because of the support and encouragement it gave him. That's when it struck me that there is a purpose for every pain.

When it came time to start dealing with the past, one of the first things that I realized is that I could turn around and find people who had gone through the same thing and help them. However, I had to be willing to let God help me in dealing with it first, so I worked through a book called, *Lord Heal My Hurts*, by Kay Arthur. It was a tough book because it really made me dig into Scripture. A lot of people would think that's boring, but if your heart is really open and you are surrendered to what God wants to teach you, you can learn a lot from a study like that. I would remind myself daily I am nothing without God. With that kind of attitude God will take you far. You must rely on him. Being able to help those people when their child was diagnosed with cancer was probably the most instrumental thing that taught my husband and I, that there was a purpose for what we had been through. There is always good in a bad situation. The suffering of my children gave me a teachable spirit.

The Bible tells us that Christ is our peace. There were a lot of times that I didn't feel very peaceful during Andrew's illness. There were also a lot of times when I felt incredible, unexplainable peace during some of the darkest times. I learned that peace really is mine in Christ and I must take possession of it by faith. Faith is simply to believe what God says, and then **act** like you believe. Waiting anxiously for that feeling of peace to come over you is not faith.

"My grace is sufficient for you, for my power is made perfect in weakness." (2 Corinthians 12:9). The Lord waited for me until I became so weak, that I was finally entirely dependent upon Him. I don't want people to feel like they are a puppet in God's hand, and I know that there is no formula to follow to come to this point of knowing God and his grace. I can only suggest that you seek a clean heart. Personally consecrate everything that you are to God. Make him the Lord of your life, and seek a personal relationship with him.

When I finally realized that relying on other people to fix things for me or come through for me wasn't working, I stopped asking people and started asking God. I didn't wait for anyone else to help me but him. I asked him to show me a way and then I had to yield to it. The peace and transformation slowly began to materialize. The verse Romans 12:2 says, "Do not conform any longer to the pattern of this world, but be transformed by the renewing of your mind..." Hannah Whitall Smith explains this verse in another book called, *The Christian's Secret to a Happy Life* she writes, "The secret lies just here, that our will which is the spring of all of our actions, has been in the past under the control of sin and self and these have worked in us all of their own good pleasure. Now God calls us to yield our wills upon Him. That he may take control of them and work in us the will to do his good pleasure. If we will obey this call and present ourselves to him as a living sacrifice, he will take possession of our surrendered wills and begin at once to work in us that which is well-pleasing in his sight through Jesus Christ, giving us the mind that was in Christ and transforming us into his image." My past had caused me to conform to a certain pattern of thinking. My mind had to be renewed so that I could begin to think in a different way. Only the love of Christ has the power to renew a mind and transform a personality.

Another verse that meant a lot to me was 1Peter 1:6-7. "In this you greatly rejoice, though now for a little while you may have had to suffer grief in all kinds of trials. These have come so that your faith--of greater worth than gold, which perishes even though refined by fire--may be proved genuine and may result in praise, glory and honor when Jesus Christ is revealed." We don't rejoice because of the suffering. We rejoice because God says our faith is "of greater worth than gold." He longs for us to put our faith in him to guide and comfort us through the suffering. He cherishes our belief in him and our willingness to ask him for help. There is a light beyond the darkness. The days will not always be so hard, so bleak, and so exhausting. It's hard to see that light when you're in the midst of dark days, but it's there. There will be a day when these present things are past and just a painful blur of memory. Make up your mind to cling to God through the darkness and let him carry you through with his mighty strength.

Whether it's overcoming temptations or going through a trial like cancer, ask God to open your eyes to understanding his spirit. Pray that God would show you who he is, and who you are because of him. I started praying that when I finally stopped rebelling against God, and I had what I feel was a spiritual cleansing. I began to experience the abundant life that Jesus came to give us on this earth. You don't have to wait until eternity to receive it. Begin your program of spiritual supplementation now, because in this world we live in, we definitely do not get enough nutrition for our souls. The love of God is the one and only pure supplement able to bring your soul to optimum health!

Resources:

We are not the only story of a cancer victim's triumph over the disease. There are many others who have tried nutritional therapy and have been successful. Dave and Anne Frahm's book, *A Cancer Battle Plan* tells of Anne's story in overcoming breast cancer that was in an advanced stage. The Frahm's book was significant not only in helping us determine Andrew's treatment, but it was the source for much of the information in our book. All quotes are attributed to the original writers and were used with permission from the Frahm's and Pinon Press. *Prescription for Nutritional Healing* by Dr. James Balch and Phyllis Balch was also essential for information on how to fight cancer. She is a certified nutritionist and he is an M.D. Both of these books should be in your home if you or a loved one are facing a cancer diagnosis. They are very inexpensive and user-friendly books.

Other recommended books:

Norman Vincent Peale, *The Power of Positive Thinking*
Carl Simonton, M.D. and Stephanie Matthews-Simonton, M.D. *Getting Well Again,*
Bernie Seagal, *Love, Medicine and Miracles*
Norman Cousins, *Anatomy of an Illness as Perceived by the Patient*
Paavo Airola, M.D. *Cancer: The Causes, Prevention and Treatment: The total approach and how to get well*
Harvey and Marylin Diamond, *Fit for life and Fit for Life II*
Wm. Fisher, *How To Fight Cancer and Win*
Max Gearson, *A Cancer Therapy: Results of 50 cases*
Harold Harper, M.D., *How You Can Beat the Killer Diseases*
Patrick Quinlan, *Healing Nutrients*

John Robbins, *Diet for the New America*
Charles Simone, *Cancer and Nutrition*
Marjorie Home, *God and Vitamins*
Bernard   Jensen,   *Tissue   Cleansing   Through   Bowel*
Management
John M. Fink, *International Directory to Alternative Therapy*
Centers for the treatment and Prevention of Cancer
Dr. William Lane, *Sharks Don't Get Cancer*

Other stories
Rick Hill Story, by Rick Hill
Cancer Holiday, by Betty Towner
Killing Cancer, The Jason Winters Story by Benjamin Roth
Smythe
How I Conquered Cancer Naturally by Edie Mae Hunsberger

Notes

Book II

Chapter 1
1. *Dayton Daily News*, August 2, 1996
2. Paavo Airola, Ph.D., N.D., *How to Get Well* (Phoenix, AZ: Health Plus, 1974), page 55

Chapter 2
1. Patrick Quillin, Ph.D., R.D., *Healing Nutrients*(Chicago, IL: Contemporary Books, 1987) page 127.
2. Virginia Livingston-Wheeler, M.D., and Edmond G Addeo, *The Conquest of Cancer: Vaccines and Diet* (New York: Franklin Watts, 1984), page 102

Chapter 3
1. Harold Harper, M.D., and Michael L. Culbert, *How You Can Beat the Killer Diseases* (New Rochelle, NY: Arlington House, 1977), page 167
2. Kurt W. Donsbach, Ph.D., D.Sc., N.D., D.C., and Morton Walker, D.P.M., *Metabolic Cancer Therapies* (Huntington Beach, CA: The International Institute of Natural Health Science, 1981), page 50
3. Ann Wigmore, *The Hippocrates Diet and Health Program* (Wayne, NJ: Avery Publishing, 1984).
4. Harold Harper, M.D., and Michael L. Culbert, *How You Can Beat the Killer Diseases* (New Rochelle, NY: Arlington House, 1977).

Chapter 4
1. Harold Manner, Ph.D., as quoted by Maureen Salaman, M.Sc., *Nutrition: The Cancer Answer* (Menlo Park, CA: Statford Publishing, 1983), page 88

2. Linda G. Rector-Page, N.D., Ph.D., *Healthy Healing* (Sacramento, CA: Spilman Printing Co., 1990).
3. Paavo Airola, Ph.D., N.D., *How to Get Well* (Phoenix, AZ: Health Plus, 1974).

Chapter 5
1. Dave and Anne Frahm, *A Cancer Battle Plan* (Colorado Springs, CO: Pinon Press, 1992) page 74
2. Harvey and Marilyn Diamond, *Fit for Life II* (New York: Warner Books)
3. Dale and Kathy Martin, *Living Well* (Brentwood, TN: Wolgemuth and Hyatt, 1988).
4. Ann Wigmore, *Hippocrates Diet and Health Program* (Wayne, NJ: Avery Publishing, 1984).
5. Frahm, page 69
6. Maureen Salaman, M.Sc., *Nutrition: The Cancer Answer* (Menlo Park, CA:Statford Publishing, 1984).
7. Mary Ruth Swope, Ph.D., and David A. Darbro, M.D., *Green Leaves of Barley* (Phoenix, AZ: Swope Enterprises, 1987)
8. Frahm, page 69
9. Max Gerson, M.D., *A Cancer Therapy: Results of Fifty Cases* (Bonita, CA: The Gerson Institute, 1990).

Chapter 6
1. William L. Fischer, *How to Fight Cancer and Win* (Canfield, OH: Fischer Publishing, 1987).
2. Patrick Quillin, Ph.D., R.D., *Healing Nutrients* (Chicago, IL: Contemporary Books, 1987).
3. Linus Pauling, Ph.D., as quoted by Lee Talbert, Ph.D., and Eugene S. Wagner, Ph.D., *Antioxidants: A Powerful Cancer Defense* (n.p.: American Institute of Health and Nutrition, 1989).
4. Dave and Anne Frahm, *A Cancer Battle Plan* (Colorado Springs, CO: Pinon Press), pages 96 and 98.
5. Dr. Bruce Miller, *Five Basic Rules for Natural Supplements*, Top 21 Lecture Tape Series, Frontrunners, 1994.

6. Joel Robbins, D.C., *Health Through Nutrition* (a self-published seminar notebook).
7. Linda G. Rector-Page, N.D., Ph.D., *Healthy Healing* (Sacramento, CA: The Gerson Institute, 1990).
8. Max Gerson, M.D., *A Cancer Therapy: Results of Fifty Cases* (Bonita, CA: The Gerson Institute, 1990).

Chapter 7
1. Norman Cousins, *Anatomy of an Illness* (New York: Bantam, 1981).
2. Richard O. Brennan, M.D., *Coronary? Cancer? God's Answer: Prevent It!* (Irvine, CA: Harvest House, 1979).

Chapter 8
1. Charles B. Simone, M.D., *Cancer and Nutrition* (New York: McGraw-Hill, 1993).
2. Richard O. Brennan, M.D., *Coronary? Cancer? God's Answer: Prevent It!* (Irvine, CA:Harvest House, 1979).
3. Dave and Anne Frahm, *A Cancer Battle Plan* (Colorado Springs, CO: Pinon Press, 1992), page 125.
4. Joel Robbins, D.C., *Health Through Nutrition* (a self-published seminar notebook).
5. Harvey and Marilyn Diamond, *Fit for Life II* (New York: Warner Books, 1987).
6. Frahm, page 132
7. Benjamin Roth Smythe, *Killing Cancer, The Jason Winters Story*, as quoted by Dave and Anne Frahm in *A Cancer Battle Plan* (Colorado Springs, CO: Pinon Press), page 132.

Chapter 9
1. Max Gerson, M.D., *A Cancer Therapy: Results of Fifty Cases* (Bonita, CA: The Gerson Institute, 1990).

Chapter 10
1. Hannah Whitall Smith, *The Unselfishness of God*
2. Hannah Whitall Smith, *A Christian's Secret of a Happy Life* (Springdale, PA: Whitaker House, 1983).

Authors

Leanne and David Sorteberg run a full-time home-based business selling the supplements they used for Andrew's treatment. Together, they share a passion for teaching others about how nutritional therapy can make their bodies healthier and their lives more enjoyable as a result. Leanne is also a licensed esthetician as well as a mother of six children. The Sortebergs reside in Burnsville, MN.

Lisa Ragsdale is Leanne's older sister. She is a full-time mother, homeschooling her four children. She and her husband, Tim, a United States Air Force officer, *currently* live in Fairborn, OH.